# GCSE Hist(

## The Schools History

Medicine Through Time
The American West, 1840-1895
Germany, 1919-1945

## Studymates

25 Key Topics in Business Studies
25 Key Topics in Human Resources
25 Key Topics in Marketing
Accident & Emergency Nursing
Business Organisation
Constitutional & Administrative Law
Cultural Studies
English Legal System
European Reformation
GCSE Chemistry
GCSE English
GCSE History: The Schools History Project
GCSE Sciences
Genetics
Geology for Civil Engineers
Hitler & Nazi Germany
Land Law
Law of Evidence
Memory
Organic Chemistry
Practical Drama & Theatre Arts
Revolutionary Conflicts
Social Anthropology
Social Statistics
Speaking Better French
Speaking English
Studying Chaucer
Studying History
Studying Literature
Studying Poetry
Studying Psychology
Understanding Maths
Using Information Technology

*Many other titles in preparation*

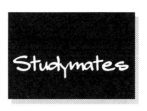

# GCSE History

## The Schools History Project

### Medicine Through Time
### The American West, 1840–1895
### Germany, 1919–1945

## Mary Kinoulty MA
Head of History, St Edmund's Catholic School, Portsmouth

www.**studymates**.co.uk

© Copyright 2000 by Mary Kinoulty

First published in 2000 by Studymates, a Division of International Briefings Ltd,
Plymbridge House, Estover Road, Plymouth PL6 7PY, United Kingdom.

| | |
|---|---|
| Telephone: | (01752) 202301 |
| Fax: | (01752) 202333 |
| Editorial email | editorial@studymates.co.uk |
| Customer Services email: | cservs@plymbridge.com |
| Series web site: | http://www.studymates.co.uk |

Printed and bound by The Cromwell Press Ltd, Trowbridge, Wiltshire.

# Contents

*Section 2: Study in depth – The American West, 1840-95*

# List of Illustrations

# Preface

This **Studymate** is a revision guide to the three most popular topics on the Schools History Project GCSE syllabus. It covers Medicine Through Time and two studies in depth: the American West, 1840-1895 and Germany, 1919-1945. It gives an overview of these units, offering a clear framework from which to revise. At the same time, it offers key details to supplement your own work. Study tips show you how to revise effectively.

**Studymates** aim to involve the student in the process of learning. There are questions throughout the book to help you check your progress and consider wider issues. Practical assignments are suggested to make revision an active rather than a passive activity. The development of the internet offers exciting new possibilities for learning. History is particularly well served by this new medium. This **Studymate** suggests a selection of web sites, to help you do research into these topics. Exploration of these sites will help to stimulate interest in the subject.

I would like to acknowledge the encouragement and practical help of my family and friends. They gave their time most generously. Without their help, this book would never have been finished. Finally, I would like to thank my colleagues and our pupils. Together, we have had a lot of fun exploring the Schools History Project.

*Mary Kinoulty*

*marykinoulty@studymates.co.uk*

# Introduction

## The structure of the course

The Schools History Project GCSE syllabus is divided into three sections:

### 1. Course work
This consists of two assignments, which vary from school to school.

### 2. A study in time
The most popular option is Medicine or Medicine through Time. This topic features patterns of change and development over a very long period of time. It is assessed by examination.

### 3. A study in depth
The most popular units are the American West, 1840-95 and Germany, 1919-45. This section focuses on a short period of time but requires detailed knowledge of the topic. It is also assessed by examination.

## How to revise effectively

The best advice is to start early, make a plan, and stick to it.

### Stage 1 – getting started
Getting started is often the hardest part of revision. Once you have started you will feel much better about the exams. The best way to stop worrying is to do something about it. Make sure that you have:

(a) a list of the topics on your particular syllabus

(b) copies of past papers to show you the type of questions set by your exam board.

*Look carefully at the list of topics*

1. Use your list of topics as a checklist for your revision.

2. Are there any gaps in your knowledge? Were you absent for any key topics? If so, sort these areas out first.

3. Which areas did you find particularly difficult? Force yourself to work on these areas at an early stage. You will feel much more confident once you have mastered them.

*Look at the past papers.*

1. How are the papers structured?
2. How many questions do you have to answer?
3. How much time do you have for each question?
4. What kind of questions are asked?
5. Which questions require document skills?
6. How many marks are allocated for each question?

## Stage 2: revising your work

**Get all your history work together** so it is easier to manage.
Consider buying **a revision file** and use it just for history.
Put your list of topics at the front so you can tick them off as you revise.
Use page dividers to help you to arrange your work in sections.
This will make revision a more manageable task.
**Highlighter pens** are useful to focus your mind on key points.

*Your best way of revising*

You have to learn the work for yourself, so think about how you revise best:

1. Do you remember what people say? If so, tape your notes and play them back to yourself.

2. Do you like using the computer? If so, word process your notes. There is a list of useful web sites at the end of this **Studymate**. It has lots of ideas to help you to increase your knowledge by using the internet.

3.  Do you find it helpful to learn from diagrams? If so, draw spider diagrams and charts to revise from. They are a good way of summing up a lot of information concisely.

4.  Are you good at making notes? If so, write clear notes either on file paper or record cards. Write in bullet points rather than full sentences.

5.  Break the task into small sections. It's better to be realistic than to be over-ambitious and then feel disappointed. Give yourself little breaks at set intervals. This will help your concentration. When you think you have learnt a section of work, ask someone to test you.

**Stage 3: last minute preparation**

Read over the relevant parts of this **Studymate** and your own notes. Do not try to cram. Just remind yourself of the key facts that you need for the exam. Remind yourself about timings and the number of questions that you have to do. Be positive. The exam gives you a chance to show how much you know!

## How to tackle the examination papers effectively

There are three golden rules when doing exams.

### Rule 1 – Follow the instructions exactly

Do the right number of questions! You will not gain any extra marks for doing more questions. You just waste time. If you do not do enough questions, you reduce the maximum marks you can achieve.

### Rule 2 – Read the questions very carefully; answer them as they are set

It is easy to misread the question. Double check that you are referring to the right source in document questions. Underline key words on the paper to help you to focus correctly on the question.

For example focus on words like 'reliable' or 'useful'. You should use these words in your answer.

1. Questions which begin with **'Why'** are looking for reasons.

2. Questions starting with **'How'** need an explanation.

3. **'How far'** in the question is a cue for you to answer on the extent to which you agree with something. You need to include words and phrases like 'completely', 'partly' or 'not at all'.

## Rule 3 – Watch the time

Be very strict with yourself to make sure that you leave enough time to answer the right number of questions properly. Write down the time that you need to start each question and stick to it. You cannot afford to get carried away on a question and then have to skimp on the rest. Write longer answers for the questions which have most marks.

## Extra advice

1. Read the whole paper through first. Choose your questions carefully. Do your best essay first. This boosts your confidence but do not get carried away with the time!

2. Write the number/letter of each question clearly in the margin.

3. Use the key words of the question in your answer. This helps to keep your answer relevant.

4. Include as much relevant detail as you can. Whenever possible include 'hard facts' to support your argument. Avoid vague general answers at all costs.

5. If you are not sure of someone's first name, leave it out. It's the surname that is important.

6. If you are not sure of the exact date, give an indication of the time frame. For example 'in the early 17th century' or 'shortly after Hitler came to power'.

7. Try to allow yourself at least five minutes to check your answer critically. See if you can spot any mistakes yourself. Save the examiner a job!

## Points to consider when answering document questions
*What kind of source is it?*
For example, is it a picture, painting, poster, extract from a letter, diary or a textbook?

*When was it produced?*
Was it produced at the time (primary evidence) or does it date from a later time (secondary evidence)? Do not assume that primary evidence is more reliable than secondary evidence.

*Note any time lapse*
For example, if someone is writing about an event a few years after it happened, they have the advantage of hindsight.

*Who produced the source?*
If you know anything significant about the person in question, include this in your answer. Is the author likely to be biased? If so, explain why but remember that biased evidence can still be useful and reliable as long as you recognise that it is biased.

*Why was it produced?*
For example, was it written simply for information purposes or was it written to justify someone's actions? Could the source be described as propaganda (information produced for a particular purpose)?

*For whom was the source produced?*
Was it meant for the general public or was it supposed to be a private communication? The intended audience makes a great deal of difference in many cases.

*Look very carefully at what you are not told about the source*
Captions like 'an eye witness' or 'in the United States in the mid-19th century' are deliberately vague. You need more precise information about the provenance (origin) of the document to make an informed decision.

1. What other supporting evidence do you need? For example, would statistics help?

2. What are you not told in the evidence? Pointing out what is missing will gain extra marks.

# Change and Continuity

*One-minute summary* – The medicine topic is a study in development over a long period of time. It is important that you understand the underlying ideas of change and continuity. Before you start revising this topic, remind yourself of the factors involved in speeding up or delaying change:

▶ the role of the individual
▶ religion
▶ chance
▶ science and technology
▶ government
▶ war
▶ communication

Remember: these factors can have a positive or negative effect. Also, any combination of these factors can be at work in any one development.

## Change and progress over time

'Change and progress over time' is the underlying theme of the syllabus. Throughout your revision, here are some key questions to ask yourself.

## Ask yourself
1. Was the pace of change fast or slow? – *Why was this?*

2. Did the rate of change vary? – *If so, why?*

3. Why did change happen when it did?

4. What factors or conditions allowed change to happen?

5. Does change always bring progress?

6. Are some developments regressive (a backward step)?

## Key factors

What does all this mean for medical development? Here are some of the key factors which helped or hindered medical development:

▶ *Religion* – played a more important role in the early civilisations, the middle ages and to a lesser extent in the medical renaissance than it does in the later period (1750 to today). Religion is a good example of a factor, which can act in both positive and negative ways.

▶ *The role of the individual* – played a greater role from the medical renaissance period onwards than it did in earlier times. This is partly because little is known about many individuals involved in medicine in the early civilisations and the middle ages. Hippocrates and Galen are important exceptions to this rule.

▶ *Chance* – must always have played a part in medical discovery as people make discoveries by trial and error. However, knowledge of this factor is limited until we have detailed written accounts.

▶ *The role of government* – became more important as time progressed. Government action became very significant from the 19th century onward.

▶ *War* – often prompts medical progress as doctors are forced to find solutions to urgent medical problems on a large scale.

▶ *Science and technology* – began to make an impact on medicine at the time of the medical renaissance. Thereafter, they become increasingly important in the development of medicine.

▶ *Communication* – also speeded up after the medical renaissance, although it had played a positive role in classical civilisations and a negative role in the Dark Ages after the break up of the Roman Empire.

## Helping you learn

### Practical assignment

Draw a grid like the one shown below. As you revise, note down examples as you recognise them.

| Period: | | |
|---|---|---|
| FACTOR | POSITIVE EFFECT | NEGATIVE EFFECT |
| Religion | | |
| The role of the individual | | |
| Chance | | |
| Government | | |
| War | | |
| Science and Technology | | |
| Communication | | |

### Exam tip

Jot down a quick list of the key factors on your exam paper. Cross it through at the end of the exam.

# 2

# Medicine in Prehistoric and Classical Times

*One-minute summary* – In this chapter you will see how medicine progressed from its earliest beginnings in prehistoric times to the fall of the Roman Empire. Look for differences between the three great ancient civilisations of Egypt, Greece and Rome. Each made a distinctive contribution to the history of medicine. The Egyptians located the major organs of the human body through their practice of embalming bodies. The Greeks started to look at natural approaches to illness but held up medicine until long after the medical renaissance by their theory of the 'four humours'. The Romans made great strides in the field of public health. Look out, too, for similarities. Knowledge of anatomy was seriously faulty in every case. Religion continued to play a major part in medicine as doctors and patients continued to place great reliance on the gods, despite the more rational teachings of Hippocrates and Galen. The pace of change was very slow. As you revise this section, make sure that you learn:

▶ what medical treatments existed in prehistoric times

▶ the key aspects of Egyptian, Greek and Roman medicine

▶ why Hippocrates and Galen were so important in ancient medicine

▶ what effects the fall of the Roman Empire had on medicine

## What medical treatments existed in prehistoric times?

There is no written evidence about medical practice in prehistoric times. Our limited knowledge is based on archaeological evidence and guesswork inspired by studying aboriginal peoples today. These sources suggest that prehistoric people could:

1. set bones

2. carry out trepanning or trephining (drilling holes in the skull). This practice was probably connected with the idea of releasing evil spirits. Medicine and magic were closely linked.

We assume that prehistoric people used herbs and plants for medicinal purposes.

▶ Question – What problems would have prevented prehistoric people from developing effective medical treatments?

The ancient civilisations of Egypt, Greece and Rome left written and archaeological evidence of their medical practices. This shows that, although progress was made in each case, ancient medicine was seriously limited.

## The key aspects of Egyptian, Greek and Roman medicine

### Egypt
In Egypt the practice of embalming corpses (making mummies) stemmed from their belief in the after life. This gave the Egyptians knowledge, but not understanding, of the body's major organs. This was an advance on the prehistoric period, as was their ability to communicate in written form.

1. The Egyptians thought that illness was caused by blocked channels in the body.

2. Their development of an effective writing system and the use of papyrus helped the communication of medical ideas.

### Greece
1. The theory of the four humours was the Greeks' major contribution to medicine. This identified the cause of illness

as an imbalance in the four humours (liquids) which were blood, phlegm, yellow bile and black bile. Treatments aimed to correct this so-called imbalance. For example, a patient said to be suffering from 'too much blood' would be bled by the doctor. These ideas persisted until the 18th century.

2.  The asclepeia (temples where the sick went to be healed by the god Asclepius) may seem ridiculous to us but they promoted a healthy life style of exercise and rest.

3.  The Greeks were thinkers rather than doers. Their system of city states did not encourage the development of medical ideas.

### The Romans

The Romans continued many of the Greek medical ideas, including the four humours. Their great contribution of the Romans lay in practical things, rather than in ideas. For example they built public health systems involving

(a) aqueducts
(b) sewers
(c) public baths
(d) toilets

in cities throughout their empire. Citizens were provided with clean water and sewage systems in a way that was not equalled until Victorian times.

The Romans also built a highly effective system of roads, which helped communication. The Roman army had well-organised hospitals.

### Remembering the similarities

Remember that there were also similarities between these ancient civilisations in their approach to medicine:

1.  They all shared a belief in gods with healing powers. The Egyptians believed in the goddess Sekhmet. The Greek god, Asclepius, was adopted by the Romans.

2.  Their knowledge and understanding of anatomy was very limited.

3. Life expectancy was short, although it was higher for the rich than the poor.

4. The Greeks and the Romans believed in the four humours.

5. Simple operations were carried out using metal instruments in all three civilisations.

▶ *Question* – How did communication help or hinder medical development in ancient times?

▶ *Question* – Was religion a positive or a negative force in classical medicine?

## Why Hippocrates and Galen are so important in medical history

Hippocrates and Galen are the two most important figures in ancient medicine.

### Hippocrates (c.460-377 BC)

Hippocrates is still known as the 'father of medicine'. He gave his name to:

(a) *The Hippocratic Oath* – This laid down guidelines for the way doctors should treat their patients. It is still used today.

(b) *The Hippocratic Collection* – This is a large number of books on medicine. We do not know how many of them he actually wrote, but the important point is that his ideas influenced medicine for at least 1800 years.

Hippocrates taught:
1. Doctors should look to natural causes of illness rather than relying on the gods. This was a very important advance.

2. The importance of noting symptoms.

3. Careful diet, exercise and rest promote good health.

Hippocrates also believed strongly in the theory of the four humours.

▶ *Question* – Do you think that Hippocrates advanced medicine or held it back?

▶ *Exam tip* – Give an overall answer to the question giving examples of how he advanced medicine and how he held it back.

## Galen (c.AD 130-200)

Claudius Galen was Greek by birth but he is regarded as the greatest doctor of the Roman Empire. He trained at the famous medical school at Alexandria. Galen was a surgeon at a gladiator's school before working in Rome for over 20 years.

1.  Galen strongly believed in the importance of dissection. He had used human bodies in Alexandria. In Rome, he had to rely on animal bodies which led to some mistaken teaching about human anatomy. However, he proved that the brain rather than the heart controlled the body by experimenting on a pig's nerves.

2.  He extended the idea about the four humours to include the theory of opposites. He said that a doctor should decide which humour was the cause of a patient's illness and should then prescribe an 'opposite' treatment. For example a person with a hot, dry fever should be given cold drinks.

3.  Galen shared Hippocrates' belief in the importance of studying a patient's symptoms.

4.  His medical books were widely read for centuries. They received the backing of the Catholic Church, which increased their influence until the reformation.

▶ *Question* – Who do you think made a greater contribution to medicine: Hippocrates or Galen?

▶ *Exam tip* – Give a clear reasoned answer, but make it clear that you know about both named individuals.

## Why Alexandria was a key medical centre in the ancient world

The Egyptian city of Alexandria was founded by Alexander the Great in 332 BC. It became a great centre of learning with a famous university and library. Dissection of the human body, which was forbidden in Greece, was allowed in Alexandria. This allowed doctors like Galen and Herophilus to make basic discoveries in anatomy.

A great source of knowledge was lost forever when this great library was destroyed by a mob in AD 391.

## The effects of the fall of the Roman Empire on medicine

The Roman Empire collapsed slowly from the late 4th century AD:

1. It split into two parts in 359 AD: the western part with its capital in Rome, and the eastern part based in Constantinople (called Istanbul today).

2. The western part of the empire was overrun by the Vandals, the Goths and other Germanic tribes in the early 5th century. In 410 AD the city of Rome itself was attacked.

3. The last Roman emperor was overthrown in 476 AD.

A long period of decline followed this collapse as western Europe slipped into 'the dark ages'. This period lasted until about 1000 AD.

### Effects of the collapse of the Roman Empire

The collapse of the Roman Empire had far-reaching effects:

1. Western Europe became increasingly lawless.

2. Communications broke down, which damaged trade and the exchange of ideas.

3. Towns were attacked and their public health systems fell into disuse.

4. Education was largely abandoned.

5. Collections of medical books were lost or destroyed.

6. The invading tribes did not value Roman civilisation.

In the general chaos, levels of health deteriorated. Doctors were no longer able to exchange knowledge freely. They lost access to medical texts from around the empire. The collapse of public health systems meant the end of fresh water supplies, sewers and public baths. This in turn left the population of towns vulnerable to disease. Europe stabilised by about 1000 AD but there was no strong government to provide highly developed communication and public health systems, such as had been in place in the Roman Empire.

This is an important example of regression in the history of medicine.

## Helping you learn

### Progress questions
1. What did the Egyptians believe caused illness?

2. What was the theory of the four humours? How did it influence medical treatment for over 1800 years?

3. Why is Hippocrates remembered today?

4. How did Galen (a) advance medicine, and (b) hold it back?

5. Why did the fall of the Roman Empire result in regression in medical knowledge?

### Discussion points
1. Which of the three great civilisations do you think made the greatest contribution to medicine: Egypt, Greece or Rome? Explain your answer. *Exam tip*: Show that you have knowledge about the other two civilisations.

2. How important was government action in improving standards of health in the Roman Empire?

## Practical assignments

1. Design your own revision table comparing the work of Hippocrates and Galen.

2. Compare medicine in the Greek and Roman civilisations. Do you think that there was more change or continuity?

3. Visit the BBC web site Medicine Through Time. You will find this a really useful site for the entire course. See list of web sites at the end of this book.

## Study tip

Make two lists:

1. ways in which Roman medicine was the same as Greek medicine

2. ways in which it was different.

Decide which you think was more important.

# 3

# Medicine from Medieval Times to the Medical Renaissance

*One-minute summary* – The main theme you should focus on in the middle ages is the positive and negative role of religion. Christianity and Islam both taught the importance of looking after the sick. However, both religions opposed dissection of human corpses, which held up medical progress. The ideas of Hippocrates and Galen continued unchallenged. The Black Death clearly showed the serious limitations of medicine in the mid 14th century. The first real breakthrough was achieved two hundred years later by the medical renaissance. Men like Paré, Vesalius and Harvey questioned the old ideas about medicine for the first time and opened up the way to a more scientific approach to medicine. However, the Great Plague of 1665 showed that medical knowledge was still very limited. To focus your revision of this section, be ready to explain:

▶ how did religion affect medicine in the middle ages?

▶ what was the impact of the Black Death?

▶ what was the medical renaissance?

▶ how did the authorities respond to the Great Plague of 1665?

▶ why did the plague die out?

## How did religion affect medicine in the middle ages?

Medicine was closely connected with religion rather than government throughout the middle ages. In the west this meant Christianity, and in the east, Islam.

## Christianity and medicine

Christianity made a major contribution to medicine in the middle ages. For example:

1. The monasteries provided the only real hospitals in Western Europe. They cared for the sick using herbal remedies. Monks even cared for lepers who were generally feared as carriers of a terrible disease.

2. The monks copied out important medical manuscripts, which had survived from Roman times.

3. The church provided the universities, which offered medical training.

On the other hand, it should be noted that the church:

(a) Actively promoted the teaching of Galen and opposed any critical questioning. People, who challenged traditional teaching, faced charges of heresy (false religious teaching).

(b) The church opposed dissection in the middle ages. This held up the understanding of anatomy.

(c) Women were not allowed to study at the universities or medical schools.

▶ *Question* – On balance, do you think that Christianity played a positive or a negative role in medicine in the middle ages?

## Islam and medicine

1. In the same period, Islam made a very important contribution to medicine in the Arab world. In particular, its influence was felt in the Middle East, Turkey, Persia (modern Iraq), North Africa and Spain.

2. The main Islamic medical centres were Baghdad (capital of modern Iraq), Cairo (Egypt) and Cordoba (Spain). These and other centres continued to use ancient Greek and Roman medical practices. Their libraries housed classical medical texts, which had been lost in the west as a result of the collapse of the Roman Empire.

3. Arab surgeons used fine metal instruments to perform an impressive range of operations including the removal of kidney stones and cataracts.

4. Rhazes (late 9th – early 10th century) was a great Persian doctor who wrote more than 200 medical books. He accurately described the differing symptoms of measles and smallpox.

5. Ibn Sina, known as 'Avicenna' in the west (980-1037), wrote the *Canon of Medicine*, which was widely read in Western Europe.

6. Islam opposed dissection during the middle ages.

▶ *Question* – In what ways could Islamic medicine be said to have been more advanced than Christian medicine in the middle ages?

## What was the relationship between eastern and western medicine?

Both Christianity and Islam taught their followers to care for the sick and the disadvantaged. Eastern and western medicine met in peace and in war. Ideas were exchanged through:

1. *Trade* – This was particularly clear at the medical school at Salerno, a port in southern Italy, where medical teachers drew on both western and eastern ideas.

2. *Crusades* – These were a series of 'holy wars' between the Christians and the Muslims, which began in 1095. The Christians were finally defeated but they had learnt valuable lessons from eastern medicine.

3. Neither western nor eastern medicine could cope with the Black Death which swept through Europe in the mid 14th century.

▶ *Question* – In what ways did Christianity and Islam adopt the same approach to medicine in the middle ages?

## What was the impact of the Black Death?

The Black Death was the greatest disaster in the middle ages. Estimates vary about the number of people who died but it is believed that at least a quarter of the population of Europe died in the pandemic (mass epidemic) of 1347-50.

Perhaps as many as one third of the population of England may have died from the disease.

The Black Death is properly known as the bubonic plague. It was spread by fleas, which carried the germs to humans from infected black rats. Victims suffered large swellings (buboes) in the armpit or groin, boils on other parts of their bodies and high fever. Most died quickly from the disease.

▶ *Project* – Find out more about the Black Death on the internet. See the list of web sites at the end of this book.

The Black Death is thought to have started in China in about 1334. It spread along the trade routes to Russia and on to Europe, 1346-49. It first appeared in England in 1348. It was particularly frightening because:

(a) it struck without warning and killed its victims quickly

(b) it affected rich and poor alike

(c) above all, the cause was completely unknown.

▶ *Question* – Why was the death rate higher in towns than in the country?

▶ *Question* – Why were the ports particularly badly hit by the Black Death?

What does the Black Death reveal to us about medicine in the middle ages? See the table on the facing page.

| Course of action attempted to treat or prevent the black death | What does this course of action tell us about medicine in the middle ages? |
|---|---|
| Toads were placed on the buboes to 'suck out the poison.' | Doctors were completely ignorant of the real cause of the disease. They did not have the necessary scientific knowledge or technology to reach the right conclusion. |
| Patients were sometimes bled in order to 'relieve the evil humours'. | The theory of the four humours was still firmly in place. |
| Flagellation. People walked in procession and whipped themselves. This was a sign of penance to show God that people were sorry for their sins. | In a deeply religious age, the Black Death was seen as punishment from God. |
| Blaming the Jews. In Strasbourg Jews were burned to death. It was believed that they were to blame. | Anti-Semitism (persecution of the Jews) was very strong. |
| Carrying of charms. | People were often very superstitious. |
| Removal of filth from the streets of London by order of King Edward III. | A connection was made between dirt and the high death rate. |

▶ *Question* – What do these actions suggest about the amount of progress in medicine between ancient and medieval times. Give examples to support your answer.

▶ *Question* – What does this tell us about the extent of medical knowledge and understanding in the middle ages?

## What was the medical renaissance?

'The medical renaissance' is the term given to the period of medical history from the mid-16th century to the early 17th century. 'Renaissance' is a French word meaning 'rebirth'. The medical renaissance is associated with the general renaissance which affected all forms of European culture from about 1450. The wider movement involved:

1. A revival of interest in classical knowledge.

2. Questioning of a broad range of old ideas. This included religious ideas, which were challenged by the reformation.

3. A more realistic style of art. Great Italian artists like Leonardo da Vinci and Michelangelo studied dissected bodies.

4. Improved communication as a result of the development of printing.

▶ *Question* – How do you think that (a) the work of artists, and (b) the development of printing might help medicine?

## Leaders of the medical renaissance

The medical renaissance involved the work of three great pioneers: Andreas Vesalius, Ambroise Paré, and William Harvey. Details of their work are given in figure 1, page 33.

You should also note the contributions of:

1. Anthony Van Leeuwenhoek (1632-1723) – a Dutchman who developed a primitive but effective microscope through which he saw microbes.

2. Thomas Sydenham (1624-1689) – an influential English puritan doctor. He encouraged the careful observation of symptoms and simple, natural cures. He wrote *The Method of Treating Fevers* (1666) and *Medical Observations* (1676).

3. Sanctorio Sanctorius (1561-1636) – an Italian scientist, who designed a method of taking the temperature of the body. However, thermometers did not become standard medical practice until the 19th century.

These medical pioneers and others made great advances in medical knowledge. In spite of this, their discoveries made little or no real difference to the way in which patients were treated with the exception of Paré's work on cauterising wounds.

| Aspect | Andreas Vesalius (1514-1564) | Ambroise Paré (1510-1590) | Sir William Harvey (1578-1657) |
|---|---|---|---|
| Background | Belgian doctor. Studied in Paris. Professor of Surgery and Anatomy in Padua (Italy). Influenced by artists who dissected bodies. | French army surgeon. Apprenticed to his brother. Later trained in Paris. Served with the French army in various wars. | English doctor. Educated at Cambridge and Padua. Worked at St Bartholomew's Hospital, London. |
| Major work | Dissected human bodies and used artists to draw them for use by medical students. Realised that Galen was wrong in important respects such as the anatomy of the heart and the jaw. | Discovered a new way of treating wounds when he ran out of boiling oil to 'cauterise' or seal them. Instead he used a lotion of natural substances. Stopped bleeding by tying silk ligatures around arteries. | Carried out experiments to prove that the heart acts as a pump, which controls the circulation of the blood. Valves in the veins prevent blood from moving the wrong way. |
| Book | The Fabric of the Human Body (1543) | Works on Surgery (1575) | On the Movement of the Heart and the Blood in Animals (1628) |
| Importance | **His work seriously undermined Galen's authority** and opened up medicine to modern medical research based on scientific dissection of the human body. | **Another challenge to traditional ideas.** Paré's methods reduced pain from wounds. The use of non-sterile ligatures could cause further infection until Lister's development of aseptic surgery. | Harvey finally disproved Galen's idea that new blood is made in the liver. Harvey did not have an effective microscope to prove the existence of capillaries. |

Figure 1. Leading figures of the medical renaissance.

Even the most respected doctors were seldom open to ideas.

▶ *Question* – What developments in science and technology were needed to make Paré's treatments really effective? *Study tip*: refer to developments in the 19th century (see chapter 4).

The return of the bubonic plague in 1665 shows that medical knowledge and understanding were still limited, despite the advances of the medical renaissance.

## How did the authorities respond to the Great Plague of 1665?

Plague had not died out completely after the Black Death. There had been periodic epidemic years such as 1625, in which plague had claimed about 40,000 victims in London.

This was eclipsed by the Great Plague of 1665 in which 110,000 died in London. The disease was not confined to the capital, but its effects were felt most acutely there because it was by far the most populated city in the country. It was dirty, over-crowded and had no effective public health system.

### The cause?
The cause of the plague was not known. It was variously blamed on a comet which appeared a few months before the outbreak of the epidemic, on stray animals, bad air, beggars, and God's anger.

### Treatments
The following treatments were used:

1. dead birds to draw the poison from the buboes

2. leeches to bleed the patient

### Warding off the disease
The following methods were employed to ward off the disease:

(a) smoking tobacco or lighting fires to clear the air

(b) carrying posies of flowers to sweeten the air

(c) carrying charms

(d) leaving London.

▶ *Question* – What do these treatments and preventative actions tell us about the extent of medical understanding in 1665?

## The action of the Lord Mayor

The Lord Mayor of London tried to contain the plague by imposing the following measures:

1. Anyone leaving London had to have an official pass and a Certificate of Health.

2. Each parish in London had to have two examiners who reported the names of plague victims to the Lord Mayor.

3. The Examiners sent surgeons and women searchers to houses, where plague was reported. They examined the sick and the dead. If they diagnosed plague, the house would be shut up. The doors would be locked and painted with a red cross and the words 'Lord have mercy on us' on it.

4. Two watchers per plague house ensured that the victims did not escape by day or night to pass on the disease.

5. The bodies of plague victims were taken away at night by cart. They were buried in mass graves called 'plague pits' in the hours of darkness and covered by quicklime to make sure that the bodies decomposed quickly. There was no funeral service.

6. Houses and streets had to be swept clean every day. Removing the dirt was the responsibility of the rakers.

7. Dog catchers were employed to kill dogs and other animals on the streets. This resulted in an increase in the number of rats.

8. Public meeting places such as theatres were closed.

▶ *Question* – Which of these regulations would have (a) helped to contain the plague? (b) made it worse? Explain your answer carefully.

The plague reached its height in the summer of 1665. Numbers of deaths from the disease fell sharply from late September until it had largely died out by the end of the year.

### Why did the plague die out?
There is no agreement as to why the plague ended in Europe at this time. Suggested reasons include:

1. The extinction of the black rat by the brown rat.

2. The improvement in public health as a result of the plague.

3. The Great Fire of London (1666) is said to have wiped out the plague in London but the fire did not destroy all the parts of the city, which had been badly hit by the plague.

▶ *Question* – Doctors in 1665 were no nearer to identifying the cause of the plague than doctors had been at the time of the Black Death. Why was that?

## Helping you learn

### Progress questions

1. How did the church (a) help, and (b) hold up, medical progress in the middle ages?

2. How did Christians learn from Muslims about medicine in the middle ages?

3. What were the main symptoms of the bubonic plague?

4. What were the main contributions made to medical knowledge by:
   (a) Vesalius (b) Paré (c) Harvey

5. What steps were taken in London to try to contain the spread of the great plague of 1665?

## Discussion points

1. To what extent had medicine in the middle ages regressed since the Roman Empire?

2. How revolutionary was the medical renaissance?

## Practical assignments

1. Design a spider diagram to show the role of religion in medicine in the middle ages. Mark the both the positive (+) and the negative (−) contributions.

2. Draw a table to compare the Black Death and the Great Plague of 1665. Compare ideas about
   (a) causes
   (b) treatments
   (c) methods of avoiding the disease.

3. Was there more change or more continuity in the response to the disease?

## Study tips

1. Remember to include both Christianity and Islam if you are asked about religion in the middle ages.

2. When answering about change and continuity, give a clear answer (say whether there was more change or continuity) but try to avoid giving an over-simplified answer. Remember that, generally speaking, some things stay the same while others change.

# 4

# Medicine in the 18th and 19th Centuries

*One-minute summary* – In this chapter you will learn how medicine began to make great strides as the result of the application of science and the gradual change in government policy. By the end of the 19th century, operations were performed with anaesthetics and antiseptics. Nursing was a respected profession and women were beginning to be accepted as doctors. Public health had undergone great improvement. At last, germs had been identified as the cause of disease and infection. A number of individuals played a key role in this period of accelerating change. In particular, you need to understand the importance of Edward Jenner, James Simpson, Joseph Lister, Florence Nightingale, Elizabeth Garrett Anderson, Louis Pasteur and Robert Koch. In order to structure your revision of this period of important change, you need to understand:

▶ how smallpox was wiped out
▶ why operations were so dangerous before 1875
▶ how operations were made safer
▶ how an effective anaesthetic was developed
▶ how antiseptics were developed
▶ women in medicine in the 19th century
▶ public health in the 19th century
▶ how the government improved public health
▶ how Pasteur and Koch found the cause of disease and infection

## How smallpox was wiped out

### The problem

Smallpox was a major killer disease. It was responsible for over 10%

of all deaths until the mid 18th century. It was highly contagious (catching). Survivors were badly disfigured by pockmarks and sometimes became blind, deaf or lame.

The story of how smallpox was overcome is popular on exam papers because it involves the combination of many factors. Revise this section in detail.

### The first attempted solution: inoculation
Inoculation involved putting pus from a smallpox sore into a cut made in the skin of a healthy person. It was hoped that a mild case of smallpox would save the patient from developing the disease badly. Inoculation was popularised by Lady Mary Wortley Montague, the wife of the British Ambassador in Turkey. Its success was hit and miss. Patients sometimes died as a result of inoculation.

▶ *Question* – Why do you think that no effective cure for smallpox had been found by 1790?

### The successful solution: vaccination
The great breakthough was made by Edward Jenner (1749-1823), a country doctor who lived in Gloucestershire. This is how he developed vaccination:

1. Jenner chanced on the discovery that people who had cowpox (a similar disease to smallpox but much milder) did not catch smallpox.

2. In 1796 he put this theory to the test by injecting an 8-year-old boy with pus taken from a cowpox sore taken from a dairy maid. The boy developed a mild case of cowpox. Jenner injected him with smallpox on two occasions but the boy failed to develop the disease.

3. Jenner repeated the experiment on other people with the same result. He had proved that giving people cowpox made them immune to smallpox. He published his findings in 1798.

4. He called his technique 'vaccination' from the Latin word meaning 'a cow'.

Jenner met a great deal of opposition at all levels. Some believed that vaccination was dangerous because it was related to an animal disease. The medical authorities tended to despise Jenner as a country doctor. Many people were simply opposed to change and were suspicious of radical new ideas. People who made money from inoculation feared the loss of their trade.

Gradually opposition was overcome. The British government gave Jenner £30,000 to open a vaccination clinic in London. In 1852 vaccination was finally made compulsory in Britain. The death rate from smallpox plunged dramatically. It was finally wiped out in Britain by the 1920s.

### Why vaccination was important

Vaccination was important because:

1. Jenner was responsible for conquering smallpox. This was man's first victory over a major killer disease.

2. The principle of vaccination was extended to other diseases. The work was continued by Louis Pasteur and Robert Koch.

▶ *Question* – What role was played by (a) the role of the individual, (b) chance, (c) scientific work, (d) the government, and (e) communication in the development of vaccination?

## Why operations were so dangerous before 1875

There was a high death rate from surgery until the late 19th century. Remember that:

1. There were no anaesthetics. The patients had to be held down. The pain was so terrible that it was only possible to perform very quick operations like amputations. Surgeons could not attempt longer, more complex, internal operations.

2. Operations were carried out in completely unsterile conditions.

   (a) Surgeons did not wear gloves, masks or gowns. They did not even wash their hands before operating.

(b) Surgical instruments were not sterilised between operations.

(c) The operating table was made from wood, which harboured germs.

(d) Bandages, dressings and sutures were not sterilised before an operation.

---

*Key tip* – Stress the fact that the underlying problem was that the doctors did not know what caused infection. Without realising it, they were spreading infection to the patients themselves and passing it from patient to patient.

---

The answer to the problem of why so many patients died from septicaemia (blood poisoning) was finally provided by Pasteur, Koch and Lister.

## How operations were made safer

There were two major breakthroughs which made surgery safer in the mid to late 19th century:

(a) The development of effective anaesthetics made operations painless.

(b) The introduction of antiseptic overcame the problem of infection.

Pain had been always been one of the most difficult problems facing surgeons. Opium and other sedatives had been used since ancient times but there was no effective anaesthetic.

▶ Project – Visit St Thomas's Hospital and the Old Operating Theatre on the internet. See the list of web sites at the end of this book.

## How an effective anaesthetic was developed

| Individual | Action | Success |
|---|---|---|
| SIR HUMPHRY DAVY English chemist | Discovered nitrous oxide vapour could be used as an anaesthetic in 1799. It was known as 'laughing gas' because it made patients laugh uncontrollably. | Its effects were very short-lived. Its use was restricted to dentistry. It was used for entertainment rather than medicinal purposes. |
| Americans including surgeon, CRAWFORD LONG and dentist, WILLIAM MORETON | Developed the use of ether as an anaesthetic, 1842-46. | Ether lasted longer than 'laughing gas' but it affected the lungs and made the patient feel very sick. |
| JAMES SIMPSON Professor of Midwifery at Edinburgh University | Pioneered the use of chloroform as an anaesthetic in 1847. He successfully tried it on himself and two assistant doctors. In a few moments they were all unconscious. They suffered no unpleasant side effects. At last a successful anaesthetic had been discovered. | Simpson soon began to use chloroform on women in labour. There was great opposition to chloroform. Pain was said to be ordained by God. Therefore, anaesthetics were unnatural. Queen Victoria helped to overcome this prejudice when she agreed to the use of chloroform when she gave birth to her eighth child in 1853. |

▶ *Question* – What did the nature of opposition to anaesthetics tell us about how people thought at the time?

# How antiseptics were developed

The development of anaesthetics enabled surgeons to attempt longer, more complex operations than had ever been possible. Sadly, this had an unexpected result. It led to more cases of gangrene and blood poisoning than ever, as the development of anaesthetics was not accompanied by any improvement in basic hygiene.

## Joseph Lister

The development of antiseptics was the work of one man, Joseph Lister. Antiseptics are substances which kill the bacteria responsible for infection of wounds.

| Joseph Lister (1827-1912) and the development of antiseptics | |
|---|---|
| Background | Worked as a surgeon (and later Professor of Surgery) in Glasgow, Edinburgh and King's College, London. |
| Work | He insisted on cleanliness during operations, proper ventilation and less over-crowding in the wards of Glasgow Royal Infirmary. This improved the situation but the death rate from sepsis (blood poisoning) continued to be alarmingly high. Lister heard that carbolic acid was being used to purify sewage in large industrial cities. He experimented with a dilute solution of carbolic acid to clean the patients' wounds (administered in spray form during the operation) and to disinfect the hands and instruments of the surgeon. This is the basis of modern aseptic (germ free) operating conditions. He was influenced by Pasteur's work. Lister showed that the use of antiseptics during an operation cut the death rate after surgery by over 30%. |
| Opposition | There was serious opposition to Lister's methods. Critics believed that the use of antiseptics slowed down operations. They said this was dangerous. The smell was unpleasant. The acid hurt the doctors' hands. Those who opposed Pasteur's work also opposed Lister's ideas. In the end Lister's work was accepted. He was given many honours for his work. |

*Question* – Why was Lister's work so important?

# Women in medicine in the 19th century

## Why were women excluded from medicine for so long?

Women had been effectively cut out of medicine since medieval times. They had no access to higher education and so they could not qualify as doctors. Nursing was also effectively closed to girls from the upper and middle classes.

1. Nursing was not considered to be a respectable profession. Nurses were generally thought to be drunk and 'unwomanly'. Nursing was restricted to the lower social orders.

2. Women from upper and middle class families did not work. Their destiny was restricted to marriage, children and household management.

3. It was considered to be unthinkable that women should have any knowledge or experience of medicine.

4. Girls' education did not equip them for a career in medicine. They learnt basic skills and 'ladylike accomplishments' like music and embroidery.

▶ *Question* – What does this suggest about the ways in which the role of upper and middle class women differed from that of working class women in Victorian times?

▶ *Question* – To what extent did the education system limit women's opportunities in the 19th century?

## Who successfully challenged these prejudices?

Three women, in particular, opened up nursing and medicine to women in the 19th century:

Florence Nightingale
Mary Seacole
Elizabeth Garret Anderson

See figure 2, page 46.

▶ *Project* – Find out more about the life and work of Florence Nightingale and Elizabeth Garrett Anderson on the internet. See the list of web sites at the end of this book.

## Public health in the 19th century

### Why did so many people die from epidemic diseases in the 19th century?

Conditions in towns in 19th century Britain were appalling. This was particularly true of the new industrial towns, which sprung up after the industrial revolution. Some of the most serious problems were:

1. overcrowding
2. no sewers; open drainage channels and cess pits
3. no fresh water supply – families had to use unreliable pumps or buy water from water sellers
4. no inside toilets – families had to share toilets which did not flush
5. poorly built houses which were cold and damp

The underlying cause of the problem was the accepted idea of *laissez-faire* ('leave things alone'). As a result nobody had any responsibility for conditions in towns. Public health was not considered to be anything to do with the government. In any case, it was generally believed that the poor lived in wretched conditions because of their own laziness and other character faults.

▶ *Question* – How did belief in *laissez-faire* lead indirectly to high death rates in industrial cities in Victorian Britain?

The death rate was shocking. This table shows the average age of death in 1842. It is taken from Edwin Chadwick's *Report on the Sanitary Conditions of the Labouring Population of Great Britain*.

| Social class | Wiltshire (a rural county) | Manchester |
|---|---|---|
| Middle class | 50 | 38 |
| Tradesmen | 48 | 20 |
| Labourers | 33 | 17 |

| Name | Early Life | Achievements |
|---|---|---|
| **Florence Nightingale,** (1820-1910). Pioneer nurse in the Crimean War, who made nursing a 'respectable profession' | Born into a wealthy family, who expected her to live a conventional life. Against their wishes, she studied at a German hospital for three months. She then ran a hospital for sick gentlewomen. | **At the request of the government, Florence Nightingale went to help in the army hospitals in the Crimean War (1854-56).** Conditions were so bad that almost half the wounded died. She cleaned the filthy wards, insisted on clean dressings and fresh air. In six months, the death rate fell to 2% of the wounded. On her return home, she wrote a government report and standard nursing books. **Florence Nightingale set up Britain's first training school for nurses at St Thomas's Hospital, London.** |
| **Mary Seacole** A nurse in the Crimean War who overcame racial prejudice and discrimination against women | Her mother was Jamaican, her father was Scottish. She nursed in the Caribbean and Central America. | **Volunteered to help in the Crimean War.** The government turned down her offer on account of racial prejudice. She went to the Crimea at her own expense and nursed throughout the war. She was given medals for her bravery. |
| **Elizabeth Garrett Anderson,** (1836-1917) Britain's first woman doctor. | Came from a comfortable home. Her decision to become Britain's first woman doctor was influenced by a meeting with **Elizabeth Blackwell,** who was the first woman doctor in the USA. Garrett is her married name. | Trained as a nurse at the Middlesex Hospital, London after failing to be accepted at any medical school. Medical students at the hospital refused to let her attend their lectures. Finally qualified in 1865 when she passed the exams of the Royal Society of Apothecaries. They did not mention women in their rules. They promptly closed this loophole. Elizabeth Garrett set up a dispensary for women (1866) and with Dr Sophia Jex-Blake, she founded the **London Medical School for Women.** |

Figure. 2 How three women overcame obstacles to pursue careers in the medical world in Victorian England.

▶ *Question* – What questions would you need to ask about these statistics to be sure that they are a reliable source of evidence?

There were many killer diseases such as:

1. typhoid – which was carried by water, milk or food
2. typhus – which was spread by lice
3. tuberculosis (TB) – spread by coughing

## Cholera
Cholera was the most frightening disease of all in the 19th century.

1. It originated in India, and reached England in 1831. There were further major epidemics in 1848, 1853 and 1866.

2. Symptoms included severe sickness and diarrhoea and high fever. Victims turned blue-grey as a result of dehydration. Victims sometimes died in a matter of hours.

3. Cholera affected people of all classes, although densely populated areas were worst hit.

4. Doctors could not agree about the cause of the disease. Theories included spreading by touch, breathing foul air associated with dirt ('miasma') or eating infected shellfish or even toasted cheese.

5. Treatments reflected this confusion. They included the application of mustard poultices to the stomach. People were advised to work hard and stay sober in order to avoid catching cholera.

> *Key point* – More than any other disease, cholera forced the government to tackle the question of public health.

## Whose actions contributed to the government change of policy?
Two figures are important to note in the field of public health at this time, Edwin Chadwick and John Snow.

*Edwin Chadwick (1800-90)*
Chadwick was a reformer and administrator; head of the Board of Health, (1848-54). He was a utilitarian. This involved strong belief

in efficiency and in the greatest happiness of the greatest number. The descriptions of conditions in the slums in his report (1842) caused outrage. Public opinion put pressure on the government to introduce public health reform.

▶ *Project* – Find out more about the work of Edwin Chadwick on the internet. See the list of web sites at the end of this book.

*John Snow*
Dr John Snow traced the cause of the epidemic in the Broad Street area of London to a particular pump in 1854.

## How the government improved public health

### The first Public Health Act, 1848
1. A General Board of Health was established in London. It had the power to set up local boards of health in any area where the death rate was 23 per 1000 or higher.

2. The local boards of health had the power to appoint a Medical Officer of Health and other officers. They had powers to insist that houses were provided with drains, water supplies and toilets.

These powers were permissive (optional) rather than mandatory (compulsory). As a result, they were not widely taken up. Chadwick was very unpopular and his enemies persuaded the government to sack him and to disband the Central Board of Health. However, this act was an important first step. It undermined *laissez-faire* ideas.

▶ *Question* – What factors led to the first Public Health Act, 1848?

▶ *Question* – The first Public Health Act, 1848, had very limited success. Does that mean that it is of no importance?

---

*Study tip* – You need to stress the principle of the act.

---

The Liberal Prime Minister, William Gladstone, introduced the Public Health Act, 1872, which divided the country into health authorities. Each had its own Medical Officer of Health but the Act did not make their responsibilities clear.

## What did Disraeli's government do to improve public health, 1874-1880?

| Act | Terms |
|-----|-------|
| The Public Health Act, 1875 | Local health authorities were made responsible for collecting rubbish, supplying pure water and providing proper sanitation. |
| The Artisans' Dwelling Act, 1875 | Allowed local authorities the power to demolish slums and replace them with new houses. |
| The Sale of Food and Drugs Act, 1875 | Clamped down on tampering with food. |
| The Rivers Pollution Act, 1876 | Banned the dumping of industrial waste and poisonous liquids into rivers. |

▶ *Question* – To what extent did Disraeli's government, 1874-80, improve conditions in the towns? *Study tip* – Think about what was done and what was *not* done.

## How Pasteur and Koch found the cause of disease and infection

By the mid 19th century, the real cause of disease still had not been discovered. Scientists generally accepted the theory of spontaneous generation, which meant that decaying material turned itself into flies and maggots. The real answer – the theory of germs – was identified by two great scientists:

(a) Louis Pasteur, a French microbiologist

(b) Robert Koch, a German doctor

## Louis Pasteur (1822-95) and the development of germ theory

| | |
|---|---|
| *Background* | French chemist and microbiologist. Pasteur was not a doctor. He was successively Lecturer at Strasbourg, Dean of the Faculty of Science at Lille University and, finally, Head of the Pasteur Institute, Paris, until his death. |
| *Work* | In his work in brewing, the wine trade and the silk industry, he found that damage was being done by micro organisms, which he called 'germs' because they were germinating or growing. They could be killed at very high temperature. This method could also be applied to milk (pasteurisation). |
| | He also saved the French silk industry from ruin caused by diseased silk worms. |
| | After careful experiments, he published his germ theory in 1861. Germs were the cause, not the result of decay. |
| | Rivalry with Koch, spurred Pasteur into further research. The French government funded his work as the German government had backed Koch. The recent war between the two countries heightened the rivalry between the two scientists. |
| | Pasteur and his team discovered a vaccination against chicken cholera using a weak solution of the germs, which had been left uncovered by accident. He used the word 'vaccine' to show his debt to the work of Edward Jenner. |
| | This principle was extended to develop vaccines against anthrax, a deadly disease, which attacked sheep and cattle (1881) and rabies (1882) |

▶ *Question* – What do you think was Pasteur's single greatest breakthrough?

# Robert Koch (1843-1910) and the fight against disease

| | |
|---|---|
| Background | German doctor and scientist who built on Pasteur's work to investigate the cause of disease in humans. |
| Work | By painstaking scientific experiment, Koch identified the germs, which cause anthrax (1878). He and his team went on to discover the microbes responsible for septicaemia (1878), tuberculosis (1882) and cholera (1883). Others used these methods to pinpoint the bacteria, which cause a wide range of diseases including pneumonia and meningitis. |
| | Koch also developed a solid medium in which to grow bacteria. The microbes were then stained purple to make them easier to study. This was much more effective than previous methods, which involved growing bacteria in liquids. |
| Assessment | Koch was a great scientist who was extremely systematic in his methods. He made great advances in the identifying of bacteria, which cause many killer diseases. He and his team of scientists were financed by the German government. |

▶ *Question* – What was meant by (a) miasma, and (b) spontaneous generation?

▶ *Question* – Why do you think that it took so long to discover the real cause of disease?

▶ *Question* – What was the role played by (a) science, (b) communication, (c) war, (d) chance and (e) government in the development of the theory of germs? Consider the work of both Pasteur and Koch.

▶ *Project* – Find out more about the work of Pasteur on the internet. See the list of web sites at the end of this book.

## Helping you learn

### Progress questions

1. What was the difference between inoculation and vaccination against smallpox?

2. Why were operations so dangerous before 1875? How were operations made safer by the development of (a) anaesthetics, and (b) antiseptics?

3. Why were medicine and nursing closed to women until the mid 19th century?

4. (a) Why was the standard of public health so poor before 1875?
   (b) What steps had been made in the area of public health by 1880?

5. What contributions did Pasteur and Koch make to medicine?

### Discussion points

1. Which factor do you think was the most important in explaining the rapid advance in medicine in this period: individual genius, government or war?

2. How successful do you think Florence Nightingale, Mary Seacole and Elizabeth Garrett Anderson were in overcoming prejudice against women in medicine in the Victorian period?

### Practical assignments

1. Find out more about Edwin Chadwick and other social reformers from the internet. See the list of web sites at the end of this book.

2. Draw a table to show the ways in which government (a) hindered and (b) helped medical change during this period.

# 5

# Medicine in the 20th Century

*One-minute summary* – Medicine has been transformed by rapid change in the 20th century. The frontiers of medicine were pushed back to limits which could not have dreamed of in earlier times. Amazing advances were made in both the knowledge and practise of medicine. The factors, which you need to stress, are war and the role of government. The two world wars speeded up progress in many areas. In Britain, the role of government took the form of the foundation of the welfare state, started by the Liberal government, 1906-14. The work was carried forward by the Labour government, 1945-51. It aimed to provide care for all citizens from 'the cradle to the grave'. The old idea of *laissez faire* had finally died. Focus your revision on these questions:

► How did the Liberal government start the welfare state?
► How did the First World War improve medicine?
► What was the standard of health between the wars?
► 'Magic bullets' the new miracle drugs
► How did the Second World War advance medicine?
► How was the welfare state planned?
► How has medicine been revolutionised since 1948?

## The position at the start of the 20th century

In 1900 there was no welfare state in Britain. This meant that the state did not accept any responsibility for the care of individual citizens. The old Victorian ideas of *laissez-faire* and self-help were still in force. There was no unemployment benefit, sick pay or old age pensions. Everyone had to pay to visit the doctor and the dentist. As a result, the health of the poor suffered badly. They *could* not help themselves and the state *would* not help them. The only alternative was the workhouse, which remained the very last resort for the poor.

▶ *Question* – Why do you think that the state was so reluctant to become involved in health and welfare?

## Why did the Liberal government lay the foundations of the welfare state?

The Liberal party won a landslide election victory in December 1905. They introduced a programme of social reform, which laid the foundations of the welfare state. This meant that the government accepted responsibility for the lives of its citizens.
The main people responsible were:

1. David Lloyd George, Chancellor of the Exchequer, 1908-15

2. H. H. Asquith, Prime Minister, 1908-16.

### Key factors
The Liberal government's social programme was prompted by many factors:

1. *The evidence of social investigations* – such as those by Seebohn Rowntree (York, 1898) and Charles Booth (London, 1891-1903). These reports showed the widespread extent of poverty. They proved that, in most cases, poverty was caused by factors such as unemployment, low pay, high rent, sickness and old age. Drinking and gambling were generally symptoms rather than causes of poverty.

2. *The Boer war (1899-1902)* – More than one third of those who volunteered to fight were medically unfit to serve. This alarmed the government since it affected the defence of the country.

3. *Sickness* – which was undermining the industrial output of the country and making it inefficient. It was feared that Britain would fall behind her rivals, especially Germany.

4. *The influence of the Fabians* – a small but influential group of thinkers who believed in gradual social change.

5. *Fear of the Labour party* – which was a threat to the Liberals as it appealed directly to the working class.

▶ *Question* – Which of these factors would you describe as (a) positive, and (b) negative?

The table in figure 3, page 56, shows the main reforms. These reforms may be criticised on the grounds that:

(a) They did not go far enough in many ways.

(b) They could be described as mean (for example, the old age pensions).

However, they are very important because they marked the end of *laissez-faire* and the start of the welfare state.

## How did the First World War improve medicine?

The First World War (1914-18) was the first total war in history. This meant that it affected every aspect of people's lives. All available resources were completely devoted to winning the war. The scale of the war was awesome. Millions of men from all over the world were involved in the fighting.

The war saw the development of new military technology. This included:

1. trench warfare
2. powerful long range guns
3. gas
4. tanks (from 1917)
5. submarines
6. aeroplanes

As a result, the scale of the casualties was appalling. In all about 1 million soldiers from Britain and the empire were killed. The number of wounded was double that figure.

| Group helped | Year | Details of the Acts |
|---|---|---|
| **Children** | 1906 | Local Education authorities were allowed to **free provide school meals for poor children.** These powers were not made compulsory until 1914. |
| | 1907 | **Medical inspections were introduced in schools.** These compulsory health checks diagnosed TB, rickets and other serious illnesses, which might otherwise might not have been detected. Local authorities could provide free medical care for children. |
| | 1908 | **The Childrens' Act** made it illegal to sell tobacco or alcohol in unsealed containers to children under the age of 16. Other parts of the act dealt with the child offenders. |
| **Old people** | 1908 | **The first old age pensions** were introduced for people over the age of 70 whose income was less than £21 per year. Single people received 5 shillings (25 p) and married couples were given 7 shillings 6 pence (37.5 p) each week. |
| **Workers** | 1906 | **The Workmen's Compensation Act** extended the 1897 Act of that name to include all workers. Employers were required to compensate workers who were injured at work. Victims of certain industrial diseases were also given the right to compensation. |
| | 1911 | **The National Insurance Act (part 1)** applied to all workers earning less than £160 per year. Each week the worker paid 4d (old pence), their employers 3d and the state 2d. In return the worker received sick pay of 10 shillings (50p) per week for 26 weeks, followed by disablement pay of 5 shillings (25p) per week; free treatment and medicines and maternity benefit. These benefits only applied to the worker not to his family. Part 2 dealt with unemployment. |

Figure 3. How the Liberals laid the foundations of the welfare state.
*Question:* what are the major limitations of these Acts?

**The effect on the medical services**

The scale of these casualties had a great impact on the medical services. Field hospitals were set up at the front. Those seriously wounded were evacuated home. Many young women volunteered to serve as nurses known as VADs (Voluntary Aid Detachments). They worked at the front and at home.

The First World War speeded up the pace of medical change. For example:

1. Blood transfusions were carried out effectively for the first time. This was made possible by Landsteiner's discovery of blood groups in 1901. Improvements were also made to the methods of blood storage.

2. X-rays were carried out as a matter of routine. This chance discovery by Wilhelm Roentgen in 1895 allowed doctors to assess the extent and nature of injuries quickly and accurately.

3. Specialist surgery was advanced. This included pioneering skin grafts and brain surgery.

4. Quinine played a valuable part in fighting malaria, which was a great risk in the trenches. This was thanks to the work of Ronald Ross, a British doctor working in India, who identified the cause of the disease as a particular kind of mosquito in 1898.

▶ *Question* – How did the First World War lead to new developments or improvements in existing medical technology?

# What was the standard of health between the wars?

**How the economy affected health between the wars**

British servicemen returning from the wars had been promised 'homes fit for heroes' by David Lloyd George (prime minister, 1916-22). Addison's Housing Act of 1919 provided a subsidy to build council houses. This was increased by the Labour government's Wheatley's Housing Act, 1924. However, these Acts did not meet the huge demand for cheap housing after the First World War.

The First World War rocked the world economy. After a short boom, there was a depression (1920-22), which was marked by high unemployment, and government cuts. Even worse was to come. The Wall Street crash of 1929 marked the start of the great depression, which lasted most of the 1930s. Unemployment in Britain reached a peak of 2.8 million in 1932. Health suffered badly in areas of highest unemployment.

The scale of the economic problems was completely new and successive governments struggled to deal with the situation.

▶ *Question* – How important do you think is the part played by housing and employment to standards of health?

## How government responded to the social and economic problems between the wars

Between the two world wars, a series of governments responded to the country's social and economic problems in different ways:

1. The Ministry of Health was set up in 1918 by the Coalition government after the devastating epidemic of Spanish influenza.

2. The Conservative government introduced pensions for widows and orphans (1925) and reduced the age for old age pensions to 65 for men and 60 for women (1926).

3. Unemployment benefit was reduced as part of the government spending cuts in response to a severe financial crisis, which split the Labour party in 1931.

4. The means test was introduced to limit unemployment benefit to the very needy (National Government, 1931)

5. Local authorities were allowed to give free or cheap milk to school children (National Government, 1934).

▶ *Question* – How effective do you think these measures were in meeting the demands of the poor during the depression?

## 'Magic bullets' – the new miracle drugs

A magic bullet is a drug which has two key characteristics:

1. It is taken internally by injection or by tablet.

2. It targets only harmful bacteria. It does not attack healthy tissue.

The first successful magic bullet was salvarsan 606, which was developed by the German biologist Paul Ehrlich in 1910 on his 606th attempt. Its significance was spotted by chance by one of his assistants. This new drug was used to treat syphilis.

Another group of magic bullets, called sulphonamides, was developed from a coal-tar base in the early 1930s. Gerhardt Domagk developed prontosil, the first breakthrough in this field. This family of drugs was found to be effective in the treatment of scarlet fever, pneumonia and other diseases. However, the greatest single miracle drug of the 20th century was penicillin.

▶ *Question* – Why were magic bullets so important in the history of medicine? Think of at least two reasons.

## How was penicillin discovered and developed for the mass market?

This is a popular question for exams. It involves the use of all the key factors in the history of medicine. Make a careful note of them as you revise this section.

It also involves an element of controversy. Alexander Fleming is popularly given the credit for the discovery of penicillin but the essential work on the mass production of the drug was the work of two other scientists: Howard Florey and Ernst Chain. All three men were jointly awarded the Nobel Prize in 1945. However, Fleming still gets more credit than Florey and Chain. As you revise, consider the question of who should be given credit for the development of penicillin.

Penicillin comes from a mould called penicillium. It was used by Joseph Lister in the 1880s but he did not exploit its potential.

The real work on penicillin was done in the 20th century when the necessary technology was available. Work was also spurred on by the Second World War (1939-45). The war not only made mass pro-duction vital; it also prompted government funding and close co-opera-tion between scientists in Britain and the United States.

## Three stages of development
Think of the development of penicillin in three stages:

| Stage | Development | Key people | Key factor |
|---|---|---|---|
| 1 | The discovery of penicillin mould | Alexander Fleming | Chance |
| 2 | The refining of pure penicillin | Howard Florey and Ernst Chain | Scientific investigation |
| 3 | The mass production of penicillin | Howard Florey, Ernst Chain, British and American scientists | War Government Technology Communication |

The three main people involved in the development of penicillin were Fleming, Florey and Chain.

*Alexander Fleming (1881-1955)*
Fleming was a Scottish doctor who worked as a bacteriologist (someone who studies bacteria) at St Mary's Hospital, Paddington in London.

While he was working as an army doctor in the First World War, Fleming realised that antiseptics could be positively damaging as they destroyed healthy flesh. What was needed was another kind of magic bullet to combat deep-rooted infection.

▶ *Project* – Find out more about Alexander Fleming on the internet. See the list of web sites at the end of this book.

*Howard Florey (1898-1968)*
Florey was an Australian doctor who won a scholarship to study in Oxford. He later became Professor of Pathology at Oxford.

*Ernst Chain (1906-79)*
Chain was a German bacteriologist also based at Oxford. Chain and Florey were brilliant scientists who worked closely together.

## Stage 1: The chance discovery of penicillin mould

Alexander Fleming made the first great breakthrough completely accidentally. On his return from holiday, he noticed an unusual pattern on a discarded petri tray. Germs were not growing around a strange mould. Clearly, the mould was killing the bacteria. A colleague identified the mould as a type of penicillium. Somehow, the name was changed slightly at this early stage to 'penicillin'.

Fleming tried to produce a purified form of the mould but had no success. He hit two problems:

1. The mould was very unstable and could not be preserved.

2. The work on purifying penicillin required chemical skills, which had not yet been developed.

Fleming found that penicillin destroyed the bacteria that cause diphtheria and meningitis. He wrote papers on his discovery in 1929 and 1931 but did no further practical work on his discovery.

▶ *Question* – What part did Alexander Fleming play in the discovery of penicillin?

## Stage 2: The refining of pure penicillin

1. Florey and Chain were inspired to concentrate on the development of a pure form of the drug by Fleming's article of 1929. It was ten years before a major team was dedicated to the work under their direction.

2. They used a variety of home-made equipment as well as using the latest technology. Even so, the process, developed by Chain, was painstakingly slow to produce tiny amounts of pure penicillin.

3. Florey successfully first tested it on mice in May 1940. The first human trial took place in Oxford in 1941. The patient started to recover but died when supplies of the drug ran out.

4. The Oxford scientists proved that penicillin was effective. The problem now was how to mass-produce the drug.

### Stage 3: The mass production of penicillin

Early in the Second World War, Florey went to the United States to ask for help from the large American drug companies. They were interested but not prepared to offer any commitment. The position was transformed when the United States entered the war in December 1941.

From then on, the American scientists joined the all-out effort to mass-produce penicillin to meet the overwhelming demand caused by the war. The work took place in the United States, where it received massive government funding. The great resources and technology available in the United States, ensured that the project was finally successful.

Large amounts of penicillin became available to allied military hospitals in time for D-Day, 1944. From then on, this wonder drug saved the lives of countless servicemen. It became generally available after the war. The first antibiotic soon dramatically reduced the death rate.

▶ *Question* – What was the role of (a) Fleming, and (b) Florey and Chain, in the development of penicillin?

▶ *Question* – What is the role of (a) individual genius, (b) chance, (c) scientific investigation, (d) war, (e) communication, and (f) government? *Study tip* – You might find it helpful to put this information in the form of a spider diagram.

# How did the Second World War advance medicine?

1. Great improvements were made in plastic surgery. This helped burns victims. Battle of Britain aircrews were among the first to benefit.

2. Further improvements were made to blood transfusion services.
3. The mass production of penicillin began.
4. Rationing ensured a fair distribution of the limited supply of food. Many people had a more balanced diet as a result of the system.
5. A free immunisation campaign was introduced to vaccinate children against diphtheria, which had a high death rate amongst children.
6. The Second World War (1939-45) affected all the citizens of Britain. Rich and poor fought together and lived through the blitz together. Everyone was fighting for a better world.

▶ *Question* – Which of these advances would have affected (a) servicemen, (b) civilians, and (c) everyone?

## How was the welfare state planned?

Sir William Beveridge chaired a government committee on the welfare system. The Beveridge Report, published in 1942, was the blueprint for the welfare state, which was introduced by the Labour government after the war.

Beveridge said that there were 'five giants' which blocked progress:

WANT  DISEASE  SQUALOR  IGNORANCE  IDLENESS

His report suggested ways of overcoming all these obstacles. His solution to 'want' (poverty) and 'disease' was an insurance scheme, which would run like this:

| *Who paid into the scheme?* | *What were the benefits of the scheme?* |
| --- | --- |
| All working people would make a single weekly payment. | A free National Health Service. |
| Their employers. | Benefits for sickness, disability, unemployment, and old age. |
| The state. | Child allowances. |

The state would care for its citizens 'from the cradle to the grave'.

### A popular report

The Beveridge Report was popular with the people as it captured the spirit of the time. It was not implemented in wartime but everything changed in July 1945 when the Labour party won a landslide election victory. The new government, led by Clement Attlee, was committed to introducing the Beveridge Report,

▶ *Question* – Why do you think that the Beveridge Report was in keeping with the spirit of the time?

*Study tip* – Think about the effects of the Second World War.

## How was the National Health Service set up in 1948?

The most difficult part of setting up the welfare state was introducing the National Health Service (the NHS). This was the job of Aneurin Bevan, the Minister of Health, who had a very forceful personality.

Under the scheme, the National Health Service offered a complete range of free medical services. These included:

1. visits to the doctors, specialists and dentists

2. eye tests, glasses and dentures

3. medicines and vaccinations

4. the services of midwives and child welfare clinics

5. ambulances

6. hospital treatment of all kinds

Hospitals were to be nationalised (taken over by the state) and run by area health boards. The NHS was paid for out of taxes and from the new National Insurance Scheme.

## How did Bevan overcome the opposition to the NHS?

*The doctors*

Many doctors opposed the introduction of the NHS. They preferred the old way of being paid fees by their patients. They did not like the idea of working for the government. A large number of doctors even threatened to boycott the scheme (refuse to operate it).

Bevan managed to win the doctors over by offering to pay them on the basis of the number of their patients. In this way, they felt that they were receiving fees rather than being given a government salary. In the end, 90% of them joined the scheme when it started on 5 July 1948.

## The problems of success

The NHS was a great success, although there were long waiting lists for the various services. The scheme was to prove much more expensive than had ever been imagined. As early as 1951, payments were introduced towards the cost of glasses and dentures. Bevan resigned over this issue. Despite these problems, the NHS remains a triumph for Bevan and the Labour Government. For the first time, good quality medical care was available free of charge to all the people of Britain.

▶ *Question* – Why did doctors object to the introduction of the NHS? How did Bevan overcome their objections?

# How has medicine been revolutionised since 1948?

The pace of medical change is increasing all the time. Amongst many other landmarks were:

1. kidney dialysis, which started in a primitive way in the 1940s

2. organ transplants

3. artificial joints

4. laser surgery using fibre optic technology

5. keyhole surgery

6. pacemakers

7. screening for cancer

8. genetic screening

9. fertility treatment

## Helping you learn

### Progress questions

1. In what ways did the Liberal government (1906-14) help (a) children, (b) old people, and (c) workers?

2. How did the First World War speed up medical change?

3. What were 'magic bullets'?

4. How did the Second World War improve medicine and welfare?

5. How was the National Health Service set up?

### Discussion points

1. To what extent was the inter-war period (1919-39) a time of regression?

2. Who really deserves the credit for the discovery of penicillin?

### Practical assignments

1. Draw a timeline to show all the main stages in the development of penicillin from Lister to after the Second World War.

2. Make a list of all the ways in which the government helped medicine in the 20th century.

**6**

# The First Settlers

*One-minute summary* – The USA is a vast country with a very diverse geography. Its interior was very sparsely populated in 1840. At that time the native Americans dominated life on the Great Plains. They had adapted their way of life to the environment. All this was to change with the growing influx of white settlers from the eastern states and Europe. You need to be aware of the differing motives for this great move west. You should also consider the difference between the myths surrounding aspects of life in the west and the harsh reality of the lives of settlers and cowboys. In order to revise effectively, make sure that you learn:

▶ the geography of the American west
▶ the early history of the West
▶ who were 'the Plains Indians'?
▶ why white settlers moved west
▶ what routes the settlers took
▶ who the Mormons were and why they moved west

## The geography of the American West

The United States of America today is a vast country with a population of 250 million. The whole country comprises over 9.5 million square kilometres.

### The Great Plains
The area of the Great Plains, which forms the focus for the study of much of the American West, extends from Canada to Texas. It is

bounded by the Rocky Mountains in the west and the Mississippi River in the east. The area has its own distinctive geography.

| Relief | Climate | Vegetation |
|--------|---------|------------|
| Wide, rolling plains with low hills | Continental climate<br>Very dry<br>Very hot summers<br>Blizzards and deep snow in winter | Grassland with few trees (the Prairie). Known as the 'Great American Desert' in the early days of the West. At that time it was considered to be unsuitable for habitation for white Americans. |

The Great Plains was home to many famous native American nations, notably:

(a) the Crow and the Blackfeet in the north

(b) the Sioux and the Cheyenne in the central areas

(c) Pawnee and the Kiowa further south.

Beyond the Rocky Mountains and the Sierra Nevada Mountains were two areas, which joined the USA in the 1840s:

1. Oregon Territory, which was British-owned until 1846.

2. California, owned by Mexico until 1848.

To the south was Texas, a large area, which became free from Mexico in 1836. Texas was an independent state until it joined the USA in 1845.

▶ *Question* – How important do you think that geography is in understanding the American West?

## The early history of the West

### Native Americans

It is believed that the native Americans have lived in North America since about 30,000 BC. They had adapted to the specific environments in the regions, where they finally settled.

## The European Americans

The Europeans first began to settle in America in the 16th century. They brought with them epidemic diseases such as smallpox, which had a devastating effect on the native Americans. One positive contribution made by Europeans to native American life was the introduction of the horse by the Spanish in the 16th century.

*The European American perspective*
From a European American point of view, the west was still largely unknown territory by 1800. Movement west became a realistic possibility when President Thomas Jefferson bought a vast tract of land from France for $15 million in 1803. This was called the 'Louisiana Purchase'.

*The mountain men*
The earliest European Americans in the west were the mountain men, who survived by hunting and trapping animals. They traded furs with the native Americans. Some, like Jim Bridger, gave valuable help to the early settlers.

*Early explorers*
The most famous of the early explorers of the far west were Lieutenant John Frémont and his scout, Kit Carson. They explored and mapped the route which was to become known as the Oregon Trail, on three expeditions between 1842-45.

Frémont's upbeat accounts of Oregon Territory encouraged the wave of settlers, who headed there later in the decade. The Mormons also benefited from Frémont's exploration of the Great Salt Lake.

# Who were 'the Plains Indians'?

## How do we know about the native Americans?

Remember that the native Americans of North America did not have a written language. This means that much of the primary source material relating to this topic comes from white Americans. There were some sympathetic observers, like the artist George Catlin, who respected the native American way of life. However, these observers were unusual.

▶ *Question* – How might the available primary sources have affected the popular image of the native Americans?

## The 'Sioux' or 'Lokota'

There were many nations who lived on the Great Plains, but the largest was the Sioux. They are often used to illustrate the way of life of the nations of the Great Plains. The Sioux prefer to call themselves the Lakota, Dakota or Nakota – depending on their dialect of the Siouan language. However, the word 'Sioux' is acceptable and is more familiar to us.

▶ *Project* – You can visit the present day Sioux nation on the internet. See the list of web sites at the end of this book.

The Sioux nation was so large that it had to be subdivided into these units:

The Sioux nation
➡
Seven tribes. The Teton tribe was the largest.
➡
Sub-tribes
➡
Bands – family groups who hunted together

The whole tribe might camp together in the summer but the bands lived separately in manageable units, each led by its own chief.

▶ *Question* – What kind of person do you think would be chosen to be the chief of the band? Why would they need those characteristics?

The Sioux nation shared a number of key characteristics:

1. They lived in tipis (also spelt 'tepees'). These were tents supported by wooden poles and covered with decorated buffalo hides. Tipis had cushions and rugs but practically no furniture because the Sioux were constantly on the move.

2. The Sioux lived a nomadic life following the buffalo, which they hunted on horseback using bows and arrows even after they had access to guns. Every part of the animal was used:

   – flesh for food including dried meat
   – fur for blankets
   – hide for leather clothes, moccasins, tipi coverings and harnesses
   – bones for tools and weapons
   – tendons for bowstrings and thread
   – horns for cups and ceremonial vessels
   – bladder or stomach for bags for carrying food and water
   – fat for soap

▶ *Question* – To what extent were the Sioux reliant on the buffalo?

## What were the beliefs of the native peoples of the Great Plains?

1. The native Americans shared a belief in the Great Spirit (Wakan Tanka) who ruled over all things.

2. They believed in the powerful spirits of the earth, the sun and the sky. All people and living creatures had spirits.

3. There was a strong belief in an after-life.

4. The native Americans lived closely in touch with their environment as a result of their religious beliefs.

5. They had a strong moral code.

*The shaman*
The shaman, or holy man, played a most important role in native American communities. Occasionally, an older married woman would be invited to take this position. The shaman:

(a) was the direct link between the Great Spirit and the band

(b) interpreted visions, which were taken extremely seriously, particularly in the lives of adolescent boys

(c) was called on to cure illness. He often had extensive knowledge of natural medicine

| | |
|---|---|
| **BIRTH** | Babies were born in their own tipis. Birth could be very dangerous. The infant mortality rate was high. The umbilical cord was preserved and kept in a special container to be treasured for the rest of the child's life. |
| **CHILDHOOD** | Children were brought up in extended families. They did not go to school. They were taught to be polite and to respect all living things. Girls and boys learnt the skills that they would need as adults. Boys went hunting with the men from the age of eight. There were elaborate initiation rites when boys and girls reached puberty. They were given adult names on the basis of visions, which were interpreted by the shamans . |
| **MARRIAGE** | Marriage took place at a young age, often the couple was aged between 12 and 15. Polygamy was common. This meant that men took more than one wife. As a result the women were protected and the men had several wives to prepare their buffalo. Polygamy also boosted the birth rate. Divorce was easy. |
| **ADULT LIFE** | Men and women had differing responsibilities:<br>• Men hunted, fought the band's enemies, and made weapons.<br>• Women – looked after the children, put up/took down/moved the tipis; skinned and prepared the buffalo carcasses; prepared the food and made clothes. |
| **OLD AGE** | Old age posed a problem because of the nomadic life style. Sometimes old people went off by themselves to die. |
| **DEATH** | Some bands buried their dead in trees or on 'scaffolds.' The dead were treated with great respect. |

Figure 4. The life cycle of the peoples of the Great Plains.

(d) played a key role in various ceremonial dances, which had religious significance. The most important was the sun dance, which required great feats of physical endurance on the part of the dancers.

## Why and how did the Sioux fight?

Bravery was highly prized by the Sioux. War gave the men of the warrior societies (fighting groups with their own customs) a chance to prove their courage. Tribes fought over horse stealing or an exchange of insults. The native Americans did not fight over land, which was seen as belonging to everyone, or take over another people. The Plains Indians had a different code of fighting from the white Americans. Their aim was to touch their enemy either in person or with a coup (wooden stick). Each warrior kept a running tally of his coups either in a coded series of feathers in his head-dress or in notches on his coup stick.

After about 1850, the native Americans were supplied with guns by white traders. However, they continued to use traditional weapons as well because they found it difficult to get supplies of bullets.

▶ *Question* – In what ways did the native Americans differ from white Americans in why and how they went to war?

# Why white settlers moved west

White settlers from the United States and emigrants from Europe began to move westward in increasingly large numbers from about 1840. The migrants had a variety of motives including:

1. *Land hunger* – The prospect of large plots of land virtually free of charge was a powerful incentive. The land in Oregon was said to be particularly fertile. Land in New Mexico was less fertile but offered great opportunities for ranching (livestock farming). Later, incentives were offered to people who were willing to farm in the Dakota Territory.

2. *Freedom* – The sense of freedom offered by a new life in the west.

3. *Jobs* – were certain in the west. The opportunities were boundless for those with initiative.

4. *Religion* – Missionaries went in search of converts. The Mormons went west to escape persecution.

5. *Gold* – was discovered in the west, sparking a series of gold rushes.

### The California gold rush
James Marshall discovered gold by chance on 24 January 1848 when he was building a sawmill on the American River. He was working for John Sutter, a Swiss immigrant, who effectively controlled California.

People joined the gold rush from all over the world. They were known as the 'forty niners' because most of them arrived in 1849. The people who made the great fortunes from the gold rush were those who supplied the miners with basic supplies at sky high prices.

▶ *Project* – There is a great deal of information about this gold rush on the internet. Visit the relevant web sites in the USA. See the list of web sites at the end of this book.

### Gold was also struck in Colorado, Nevada and Montana (1859-60)
The discovery of gold in the hills of South Dakota in 1874 was to spell disaster for the Sioux. They considered those hills to be sacred. The conflict over the mining rights led directly to a revival of the Indian Wars.

### Government policy
The United States government encouraged the move west. It was anxious to extend its territory into these remote areas.

▶ *Question* – Why do you think that (a) a poor person from England or Ireland (b) a poor farmer from the eastern states of America might have been tempted to move west? Give several reasons. *Study tip*: think about the positive (what attracted them?) and the negative forces (what were they escaping?)

## The routes the settlers took

There were many routes overland but the most important were various trails.

### The trails

1.  The Oregon Trail – a 2,000 mile route over the Rocky Mountains from Independence and other 'jumping off points' in Missouri to the rich farmland of Oregon. The first pioneers arrived in 1836 but the great migration started in 1843. It was used by about 500,000 people before it was overtaken by the opening of the transcontinental railroad in 1869.

2.  The California Trail – followed the Oregon Trail from Missouri to Idaho, where it branched off to California.

3.  The Mormon Trail – went from Illinois to Salt Lake City, Utah Territory. It used part of the Oregon Trail. The Mormons' great organisational skills helped other travellers.

4.  The Santa Fe Trail – went south from Missouri to Santa Fe, New Mexico. It involved crossing desert lands. It provided access to the southern ranches until the arrival of the railroad in the 1880s.

▶ *Question* – Which trail would have been used by those looking for (a) farmland, (b) cattle ranching, and (c) gold ?

▶ *Project* – Visit the Oregon Trail site on the internet. You can find lots of fascinating details about life on the journey. See the list of web sites at the end of this book.

### What were conditions like on the trails?

The pioneers travelled in covered wagons. These had iron wheels, which made the journey rough and uncomfortable. The wagons were sometimes so heavily laden that many people had to walk most of the trails on foot. People travelled in large groups led by a wagon captain. Rules were agreed in advance.

## Dangers

The wagon trails posed many dangers including:

▶ *Disease* – 1 in 10 people died on the Oregon Trail generally from disease. Cholera was particularly dangerous. There was no real medical help available.

▶ *Accidents* – Children often fell under the wagon wheels. There were also accidents with guns.

▶ *Crossing rivers* – People and animals were drowned, and wagons and supplies were damaged or lost.

▶ *Running out of food and drink* – Water was scarce particularly on the Santa Fe Trial. Prices rose as supplies became harder to obtain.

▶ *Terrible storms* – These were particularly dangerous on the plains as there was no shelter. Wagons stuck in the mud.

▶ *Resources* – Later migrants had problems with shortages of buffalo 'chips' (dung used as fuel for fires), and wild life. This was because supplies had been used up by those who had gone before them.

▶ *Attacks from Indians* – This was often the pioneers' greatest fear. In fact the Indians were often helpful and friendly particularly in the early days. More pioneers died from disease than from Indian attacks. Attacks took place as the migrants became seen as an increasing threat.

*Example – the Donner Party*
The dangers of the wagon trails were frighteningly demonstrated by the Donner Party. This group took what they thought was a short cut on the final stage of their journey to Sutter's Fort (now Sacramento), California. They got trapped in the Sierra Nevada Mountains in the terrible winter of 1846-47. The 47 survivors out of the original party of 81 had resorted to cannibalism.

▶ *Question* – What preparations do you think that people should have made before starting out on a wagon trail?

## Who were the Mormons and why did they move west?

One of the earliest movements west by white settlers was that of the

Mormons. The Church of Jesus Christ of the Latter Day Saints, as it is properly called, was founded by Joseph Smith with six members in 1830.

Smith said that, as a boy of 14, he had been led by an angel called Moroni to find gold plates buried in a hillside near his home in Palmyra, in New York State. After translating the secret inscriptions on these plates, he published the *Book of Mormon* (1830) which reveals the beliefs of the church.

### Mormon beliefs

The Mormons differed from the Christian churches in many important areas of belief. They were also set apart by their distinctive church organisation and style of worship, which took place in a temple rather than in a church. Above all they were treated with suspicion because of their practice of polygamy in the early days.

Suspicion and fear of the unknown soon led to violent persecution of the Mormons. In response, they moved steadily west until they reached their final destination in Salt Lake Valley in 1847. The main stages of their migration west are shown in figure 5, page 78.

▶ *Question* – Why do you think that the Mormon Trail was so successful?

## Helping you learn

### Progress questions

1. Who were (a) Jim Bridger, (b) John Frémont, and (c) Joseph Smith?

2. Why was the buffalo so important to the Sioux nation?

3. What were the differing roles of Sioux men and women?

4. How do you explain the upsurge in the population of Oregon and California in the 1850s? *Exam tip*: Be as exact as you can in your explanation. For example, give factual details about the discovery of gold at Sutter's Mill in 1848.

5. What dangers did the pioneers face on the long distance trails?

6. Why did the Mormons move west? What was their route?

| Place | Date | Detail |
|---|---|---|
| **Kirtland,** Ohio | 1831-38 | **The Mormons' first major settlement**. Relations with the 'gentiles' (non Mormons) became increasingly difficult. Mormons were often attacked and their property burnt. The same pattern was followed in another Mormon colony near Independence, Missouri. The last straw was the collapse of the Mormon Bank in 1837. The Mormons were unfairly blamed by people who had lost money. **They moved further west.** |
| Commerce (renamed **Nauvoo**), **Illinois** | 1838-46 | **Joseph Smith** took over the small settlement of Commerce, which they re-named Nauvoo. There were many converts. By 1842, Nauvoo was a leading town in Illinois. However, trouble continued. **Joseph Smith and his brother, Hyrum, were killed by a mob** in 1844. **Brigham Young took over as leader.** He decided to lead 'the saints' to the **New Jerusalem in the west** where they need have no contact with hostile 'gentiles'. |
| **Salt Lake City** (Mexican territory until 1848; Utah did not join the USA until 1896 after polygamy was banned in 1890) | 1846 – present | **Brigham Young led some 1,600 Mormons on an epic journey west to the Great Salt Lake**. He planned every aspect of the journey including the daily timetable. The route was scouted ahead of the main party, which was divided into companies with captains and sub-captains. In spite of all this planning, they still suffered hardship and disease. The Mormons spent the terrible winter of 1846-7 in Winter Quarters (Nebraska). In spring 1847 Brigham Young led an advance party of 143 men, 3 women and 2 children to the Great Salt Lake. **They arrived in July 1847** and transformed it from a desolate spot into a thriving self-supporting community. |

Figure 5. The main stages in the Mormons' move west.

## Discussion points

1. The old western films tended to show the 'Indians' in a very poor light and the settlers in a very romantic light.

   (a) Why do you think this was the case?

   (b) Do you think that modern films paint the same kind of picture?

2. Why do you think the Mormons provoked so much opposition?

## Practical assignments

3. Draw a spider diagram to show differing aspects of Sioux life. Include tipis, hunting, warfare, religion, and family life.

4. Carry out further research on the native Americans on the internet. See the list of web sites at the end of this book. Individual nations have their own web sites so you can hear their history at first hand.

# 7

# Settlement and Conflict in the West

*One-minute summary* – After the first great wave of settlers was over, the new arrivals had to carve out a new life for themselves in the west. The old westerns paint an exciting picture of life in the west. There was much excitement and opportunity but life was very hard for many people. This raises one of the themes of this section: the contrast between myth and reality. The other great theme that you must consider is that of conflict. The tension between the native Americans and the new settlers came to a tragic conclusion with the Massacre at Wounded Knee, 1890, which saw the final defeat of the native Americans. They lost their right to live freely according to their own traditions forever. In order to explore these themes, you need to investigate:

▶ the lives of farmers and women on the Great Plains
▶ the impact of the new railroads on daily life
▶ the realities of cowboy life
▶ law and order in the 'wild west'
▶ why relations broke down between native and white Americans
▶ the impact of defeat on the lives of the native Americans

## The lives of farmers and women on the Great Plains
### The 'homesteaders'
Technically, 'homesteaders' were farmers who benefited from the Homestead Act, 1862. Its aim was to make land available land to poor farmers in sparsely populated states. The aim of Abraham Lincoln's policy was to:

1. settle the sparsely populated interior with farmers
2. prevent speculators (people who take a financial risk to make a great profit) from cashing in.

*The Homestead Act, 1862*
1. ...allowed a man over 21 or head of a family to take 160 acres of land, which had been surveyed by the government. In order to own the land officially, the homesteader had to cultivate the farm for five years. They had to pay a $10 fee. The speculators still managed to cash in but the act was very successful overall.

2. Homesteaders could double their holding by claiming another 160 acres of land provided they planted 40 acres with trees under the terms of the Timber Culture Act, 1873.

The Desert Land Act, 1877 offered government grants of 640 acres of land in very arid areas provided that irrigation work was undertaken.

▶ *Question* – Why do you think that the government was prepared to give so much free land to farmers?

*What was life like as a homesteader?*
Getting the land was only the start of a homesteader's problems. Building a house was very difficult in a region where there were no trees and very little access to timber before the railroad arrived. The solution was the 'sod house', which was a house built from sods, which were cut from the topsoil of the prairie.

*Hard farming*
Farming often proved to be unexpectedly difficult on the prairies. Newcomers from the eastern states, or Europe, generally had farming experience. This was largely irrelevant on the vast treeless plains, which suffered terrible extremes of climate. Farmers eventually found the solutions to their problems by learning to adapt to their new environment. See figure 6, page 82.

## What was life like for women on the Great Plains?

Life was often very hard for women. They had to make homes and bring up their families in very difficult circumstances a long way from home. There were no local shops. They had to make do with what was to hand. Women collected buffalo 'chips' (dung) for fuel.

| Problem | Solution |
|---|---|
| **Cultivating the vast areas of the prairies** by hand was too slow. | **The steel plough** was developed by John Deere in 1837. It was in common use in the prairies by the 1850s.<br>**A horse-drawn reaper** was patented by Cyrus McCormick in 1831. It could cut 12 acres of corn per day. It revolutionised farming on the prairies.<br>**Horse-powered threshing machines** were developed in the 1840s to separate the grain from the stalk, which had been a long process done by hand. |
| **Animals trampling crops.** | The development of **barbed wire**, invented by Joseph Glidden in 1874. |
| **Plagues of grasshoppers** destroyed entire crops, particularly in Dakota, 1874-77 | Farmers planted wheat earlier and experimented with other crops.<br>**Insecticides** were developed in the 1890s. |
| **Lack of water.** This was extremely serious as there were no lakes and very few rivers and droughts were common in the summer. | **Dry farming.** A method of farming with very little water. It involved: ploughing the land every time in rained; using 'dust mulches' which did not allow the rain to evaporate and changing to more appropriate crops.<br>**Wind pumps.** Farmers dug deep wells often by hand. The water was raised to the surface by wind power. They became a common sight all over the prairies. |

Figure 6. The problems faced by farmers on the Great Plains, and how they solved them.

They cooked using unfamiliar ingredients, fetched water, and made clothes. Many women helped with ploughing, building houses and other traditionally male tasks.

*Health and sickness*
Women had a major role looking after family members who were sick or injured. There was a dire shortage of doctors and midwives. Women had to give birth with little or no help. There were no hospitals in the early days of the west. As a result, women often died in childbirth. There was also a high death rate among babies and children.

*'School marms'*
Women could become school teachers. They were known as 'school marms' (short for 'madams'). They were generally well-respected but badly paid.

▶ *Question* – In what ways did women contribute to life on the Great Plains?

## The impact of the new railroads on daily life

The great improvement in communications transformed life in the west. See figure 7, page 97. The greatest impact was made by the railroad. The opening of the transcontinental route in 1869 started a wave of railway building in the west.

▶ *Project* – Find out more about the Pony Express and Wells Fargo on the internet. See the list of web sites at the end of this book.

### Effect of the new railroads
This upsurge in railroad building had far-reaching effects on life in the west:

1. *Newspapers* – were able to increase their circulation thanks to the railroad.

2. *Boom towns* – sprang up along the mainline routes. Towns without easy access to the railroad often went into decline.

3. *Diet* – improved, as it was now easy to bring in food from long distances.

4. *Farming* – Farmers could buy agricultural machinery, seeds and fertilisers in bulk, and send their crops to the coast for export abroad.

5. *Supplies* – Homesteaders could buy wood and other building materials.

6. *The new industries* – could buy essential raw materials from the north and east and reach mass markets to sell their manufactured goods.

The native Americans were alarmed by the rapid growth of the railroad. They realised that it was a threat to their way of life.

▶ *Question* – Which were (a) the positive results, and (b) the negative results of the coming of the railroad?

▶ *Question* – In what ways did the railroad pose a real threat to the native Americans?

## The realities of cowboy life

### Who were the real cowboys?
The cowboys are an essential part of the folklore of the west. Their job was to look after the cattle for the ranch owners and to drive great herds on long trails. They rode in set formations designed to ensure that they did not lose any of the animals. The trail master was in charge.

A significant proportion of American cowboys was black or Mexican. They were strong and skilful but poorly paid.

### Cowboy clothes
Cowboys dressed in a way to suit their job:

7. a large hat to shade them from the sun or protect them from the rain

8.  high heeled boots to make sure that their feet stayed in the stirrups

9.  tight pants (trousers) with leather 'chaps' to prevent chafing and to keep out insects and dust

10. a bandanna (handkerchief) tied at the neck could cover the nose and mouth in case of dust clouds

They were very skilled horsemen. They were expert with the lasso, which was used when a cow needed to be branded. This was a recognised symbol applied to every animal in the herd with a hot branding iron. It was done so that the cowboys knew who owned which animals. The aim was to make cattle rustling (theft of cattle) more difficult.

▶ *Question* – Why do you think that a cowboy's life seemed glamorous to people living in the eastern states?

▶ *Question* – How glamorous do you think that the cowboy's life was in reality?

Study tip: give details of the problems that the cowboys faced.

### The cattle drives north from Texas

In the 1830s, cattle ranching on a large scale was limited to Texas, where the great cattle barons owned huge herds. The great drives north did not begin until after the American Civil War (1861-65). The Texas ranchers realised that they could sell their livestock in the great northern and eastern cities for up ten times the price that they would reach at home.

The solution was to use cowboys to drive their herds north to a convenient railhead (a railroad station) from where they could be sent by train to the big cities. Cattle drives of 2,000-3,000 head of cattle were common.

*The main routes included:*

(a) The Chisholm Trail to Abilene in Kansas. This was the first major 'cow town' (a railhead from where cattle could be sent by railroad to the major towns in the east). It was developed by Joseph McCoy.

(b) The Goodnight-Loving Trail, which went through New Mexico and Colorado to Wyoming. It was developed by the great cattle baron, Charles Goodnight and his partner, Oliver Loving. It involved crossing desert areas and passing through Comanche territory.

The cattle drives were unsatisfactory in the long run because:

1. The cattle suffered on the long trails. There were always losses.

2. Only tough long horn cattle were strong enough to survive the drives. The cities were looking for better quality meat.

### The development of ranching on the Great Plains

This was the logical solution to the problems associated with the long cattle drives. Charles Goodnight led the way by buying a ranch in Colorado in 1870. He stocked it with cattle from his base in Texas. Ranching soon spread across the plains. States like Wyoming, Kansas, Dakota and Colorado saw the growth of huge ranches. The most famous of the new cattle barons on the Great Plains was John Iliff, who started ranching in Colorado with a herd, which he bought from Goodnight and Loving. He later extended his ranching business to Wyoming.

*Problems of open ranching*
At first the cattle roamed free, identified only by their distinctive brands. This led to problems such as:

(c) disease spread easily among the cattle

(d) cattle rustling was common

(e) selective breeding was impossible

Not surprisingly, there was conflict between the ranchers and the homesteaders, as there was a clash of interests over the land. The homesteaders used the new invention of barbed wire to fence in their land and protect their farms from the free-range cattle. The ranchers hated its use because it blocked their access to water.

*The worst conflict*
The worst example of conflict between ranchers and farmers was the 'Johnson County War', which broke out in Wyoming in 1889. The cattlemen resented the homesteaders, who began to arrive in the early 1880s. The terrible winter of 1886-87 highlighted the difficulties between the two sides. Relations got steadily worse. The first victims of the 'war' were Jim Averill and his partner Ella Watson, who was said to have been involved in cattle rustling. They were lynched (killed without a trial) by a gang led by a local cattle rancher in 1889.

*Hired guns*
The number of killings mounted as the cattle barons brought in hired gunmen, many of whom came from Texas. The violence was at its height in 1891 and 1892. The worst incident was a shoot out at the KC Ranch in 1892. In the end, the army restored order. The Texan gunmen were treated very leniently by the authorities.

*Peaceful living*
Ranchers and homesteaders gradually came to live together peacefully. The ranchers came to realise the benefits of the hated barbed wire. Its use allowed them to crossbreed their Texas long horn cattle with imported cattle like Hereford bulls from England. This resulted in better quality meat and more milk. The new breeds could not withstand the long drives. The days of the great cattle trails were over.

*Technology*
The ranchers also used wind pumps to allow them to water their cattle in the driest area.

▶ *Question* – How did the cattlemen adapt to (a) changing conditions and (b) improved technology?

# Law and order in the 'wild west'

## How wild was 'the wild west'?

The Johnson County war highlights the popular image of the 'wild west'. We get the impression from old western films that gunfights were common, and that innocent people went in fear of their lives. How true is this picture?

The really 'wild' behaviour was largely confined to:

1.  The gold fields, where there was serious trouble over claims and theft. Miners' Committees tried to maintain order but as the situation deteriorated vigilantes enforced lynch law in the absence of a properly organised legal system. This meant hanging offenders without a trial.

2.  The cow towns such as Abilene and later Dodge City, Kansas. After three months or more on the cattle trail, cowboys arrived in these towns ready to let off steam. The combination of pay, drink and gambling could easily lead to violence. However, these towns also had many citizens, who wanted a peaceful life. In Abilene, they were supported by Marshal Thomas Smith, who enforced the law fearlessly until he was murdered in November 1870. Abilene was overtaken by Dodge City and other cow towns. Ordinary life continued despite outbreaks of violence.

## Colourful characters

There were many colourful characters in the west. These include:

1.  *Outlaws* – like Billy the Kid (real name possibly William H Bonny) who was said to have committed his first murder at the age of 12 and Jesse James. He and his gang robbed banks, trains and stage-coaches. He was shot by a gang member, who wanted to claim the reward.

2.  *Lawmen* – like Wyatt Earp, Marshal of Dodge City in its wild days. He is famous for the shoot out at the OK Corral, in which he and his brothers and 'Doc' Holliday killed members of the Clanton gang, in Tombstone, Arizona. Accounts and opinions about what really happened vary significantly.

3. *Larger than life personalities* – like 'Calamity Jane' (real name Martha Jane Canary). She defied the conventions of the day by fighting, drinking and wearing men's clothes. She claimed that she lived with 'Wild Bill' Hickok (real name James Butler) until he was killed in Deadwood, now in South Dakota. This claim is now thought to be unlikely. She later she joined Buffalo Bill's Wild West Show.

It is important to take many of the stories with a pinch of salt. People like Calamity Jane liked to exaggerate their own life stories. The story of Billy the Kid was first told by his killer, Pat Garrett. The number of really ruthless gunmen in the 'wild west' was probably much lower than we would imagine.

▶ *Project* – Find out more about these and other colourful characters by looking them up on the internet. See the list of web sites at the end of this book.

### Taming the wild west

The west was gradually tamed by a number of factors:

1. the decline of the long distance cow trails and cow towns

2. the development of fast communications helped the forces of law and order, as the west became less remote (see figure 7, page 97)

3. the spread of federal government as the western territories were accepted into the Union. Statehood involved a clearly defined State government with links to the federal government in Washington. There was a clear system of law administered by marshals in towns and sheriffs at the county level.

## Why relations broke down between native and white Americans

### What caused the 'Indian Wars'?

The most tragic conflict in the American West was between the native Americans and the white settlers, who had been steadily taking over their traditional hunting grounds. Tensions rose dramatically with the Californian gold rush, and the increasing movement west by the settlers.

▶ *Question* – The native Americans and the white settlers had completely different ideas about land ownership. What were they?

▶ *Question* – Do you think that the Indian Wars were inevitable (bound to happen)?

## The attempt at a peace settlement

The Fort Laramie Treaty of 1851 was the government's attempt to reach a peace settlement:

| *What the Indians gained* | *What the Indians gave up* |
|---|---|
| Both sides agreed to 'lasting peace'. The US government promised to protect the Indians. | They accepted the government's right to build roads and military posts. |
| The US government agreed to pay the Indians $50,000 each year for ten years. | The major native American nations were allocated areas where they would live, although they did not give up their claims to other lands. |
| Possibly payment in kind (such as farming tools) might be made for a further five years. Payment could be stopped to any nation which broke the treaty. | |

The areas set aside for the Indians were generally of poor land, well away from the trails. The nations were split up to reduce their potential threat to the settlers.

▶ *Question* – Why was this treaty in the government's favour?

▶ *Project* – Look up the exact terms of the this treaty on the internet. See the list of web sites at the end of this book.

## How was peace broken after the Treaty of Laramie, 1851?

Conflict continued with provocation on both sides. Notable flash points include:

1. Grattan's Massacre, 1854. Lieutenant Grattan opened fire on a Sioux band following a misunderstanding over a cow. This attack provoked war.
2. The discovery of gold in the Colorado Mountains (1859) brought waves of white people to land, which had been assigned to the Indians.
3. The Sand Creek Massacre (29 November 1864). This terrible massacre was carried out by a volunteer force commanded by Colonel John Chivington. They attacked a peaceful encampment of more than 450 Cheyennes and Arapahos led by Chief Black Kettle. They had been legally settled in the barren area of Sand Creek in Colorado Territory. A US government committee condemned the massacre but the basic policy remained unchanged. The southern nations were bribed and threatened into agreeing to move into reservations in Oklahoma.
4. The Bozeman Trail caused another upsurge in the on-going conflict. This route was pioneered by John Bozeman to open up the Montana gold fields. It antagonised the Sioux because it crossed their prime hunting ground, the Little Big Horn area. The authorities built three forts to protect the road. This made the situation even worse.
5. The Fetterman Massacre (21 December 1866). The Bozeman Trail provoked Chief Red Cloud to take revenge on the soldiers. The victims were a party of 80 soldiers from Fort Philip Kearny led by Captain William J. Fetterman, a reckless, over-confident officer who hated Indians. The entire party was killed by a force of Sioux, Cheyenne and Arapoho warriors.

▶ *Question* – To what extent did the white authorities provoke the conflict with the Indians in the period 1859-66?

## How did the government change its policy?

Relations between the white authorities and the Indians were at an all time low. Clearly, a new approach was needed. A new government commission decided that the answer lay in small, scattered, reservations, where the Indians would be taught to adopt the white way of life.

▶ *Question* – What do you think was the real purpose behind this new policy?

The Medicine Lodge Council (Kansas), 1867, attempted to enforce this policy on the nations of the southern plains with some limited success. The Fort Laramie Treaty was concluded with the northern nations the following year.

### The Fort Laramie Treaty, 1868

| What the Indians gained | What the Indians gave up |
|---|---|
| The Bozeman trail and the forts along the route were abandoned. | The Sioux and other northern nations agreed to settle in a reservation in Dakota. They were to be given individual grants of land. They were to be taught to farm. |
| The Sioux were allowed free access to the Little Big Horn hunting grounds. White people were not to settle in this area without the permission of the Indians. | The Indians agreed not to oppose any more railroads or wagon roads. |

▶ *Question* – Was this treaty more or less favourable to the Indians than the First Treaty of Fort Laramie, 1851?

▶ *Project* – Find the exact terms of this treaty on the internet. See the list of web sites at the end of this book.

It looked as if peace was finally in sight. President Ulysses S. Grant and his supporters favoured an Indian Peace Policy based on encouraging the Indians to adopt the white way of life. They could not see that they were imposing an alien way of life on the native American people.

In any case, key army officers did not share the ideas of the Indian Peace Policy. General Philip Sheridan, General William Sherman and Lieutenant-Colonel George A. Custer believed that the only answer to the conflict was to wipe out the Indians.

The Massacre at Washita River 1868 was the killing of over one hundred Cheyennes and Arapahos who were peacefully encamped by the Washita River. Most of the victims were women and children. Their leader was Chief Black Kettle. He and his wife were killed. The attack was led by Custer, who was a very controversial officer.

## What led to the Battle of the Little Big Horn, 1876?

More serious trouble was sparked by the discovery of gold by Custer's men in the Black Hills of South Dakota in 1874. The government tried to buy the land from the Sioux but no agreement was reached. Prospectors and settlers poured into the area, provoking the anger of the Sioux. Many left the reservations.

*More tension*

The government escalated the tension by ordering all Indians to return to the reservations by 31 January 1876. Sitting Bull and Crazy Horse refused. Others did not even know about the order. The stage was set for war.

The Sioux gathered along the Rosebud River in modern day Montana. They were joined by Arapaho and Cheyenne bands, who believed there was safety in numbers. General Sheridan decided to surround and kill them.

*The attack*

There was to be a three-pronged attack led from different directions by:

1. General Crook
2. Colonel Gibbon
3. General Terry and Lieutenant-Colonel Custer, who was in disgrace. Custer had been court-martialled twice and was unpopular with his men.

General Crook was beaten back by superior numbers on 17 June 1876. The Indian chiefs moved their camp to the Little Big Horn hunting grounds, where they were tracked by US army scouts. Gibbons and Terry planned an attack involving Custer. He was given written orders from General Terry but he disobeyed them. He chose to attack without waiting for Colonel Gibbons.

▶ *Project* – Find the exact text of Terry's orders to Custer on the internet. See the list of web sites at the end of this book.

## What happened at the Battle of the Little Big Horn, 25 June 1876?

Custer divided his force into three sections. He commanded one.

Major Reno and Captain Benteen were to command the other two groups.

Custer had completely underestimated the size and strength of the opposing force. He was surrounded by a huge force of well-armed Indian warriors led by Chiefs Red Cloud and Sitting Bull. Custer and his entire force of over 200 men were killed. Reno and Benteen were powerless to help. They were pinned down on a nearby hilltop by overwhelming numbers.

'Custer's Last Stand' is one of the most controversial events in the Indian Wars. His supporters present him as a hero. To his critics, Custer was an ambitious man, bent on gaining glory and promotion.

*Backlash against the Indians*
There was a terrible backlash against the Indians in the wake of the Battle of the Little Big Horn. They were forced back to the reservations. Chief Sitting Bull led his people to Canada, where they stayed until 1881. Crazy Horse was captured and killed by a soldier in 1877.

▶ *Question* – Why was Custer defeated at the Battle of the Little Big Horn?

▶ *Question* – Why is it difficult to find out exactly what happened at this Battle?

▶ *Project* – Find out more about Custer and Sitting Bull on the internet. See the list of web sites at the end of this book.

## What led to the Battle of Wounded Knee, 1890?
The spirit of the Indians had been broken in the aftermath of the Battle of the Little Big Horn. However, they found new inspiration in the ghost dances. These were special dances in honour of the Great Spirit. The dancers wore special 'ghost shirts' covered with symbols, which they thought would protect them from white men. The dancers were told that they would bring about the return of their lost lands and dead warriors. The US authorities were alarmed by the ghost dances, which they did not understand. They determined to stop them.

*The shooting of Chief Sitting Bull*
Chief Sitting Bull was wrongly thought to have encouraged the ghost dances. He was shot and killed by Reservation Police who came to arrest him at his home at Standing Rock, 15 December 1890.

*A massacre*
This prompted Chief Big Foot to move his band to join Red Cloud at the Pine Ridge Reservation. They were stopped by part of the 7th Cavalry and brought to the army post at Wounded Knee Creek.
The next day, 29 December 1890, the soldiers searched their prisoners for weapons. In the ensuing confusion, a gun was fired. This triggered a great outbreak of shooting, in which more than 200 Indian men, women and children were killed. Those who escaped, died in the snow. The 'battle' was, in fact, a 'massacre'.

## The end of the Indian Wars
Wounded Knee marked the end of the Indian Wars. The Indians were forced back to their reservations, where they were compelled to adopt the culture of the white men. Under the terms of the Dawes Act, 1887, they had been given individual grants of land. However, many did not want the land and sold it for small sums. This left a large surplus of land in Oklahoma. It was given to white settlers in land races starting in 1889. This met the demand for more land by would-be settlers.

## Life on the reservations
The life of the Indians on the reservations was utterly miserable. As planned, they became increasingly dependent on their white masters. They never adapted to farming. The children were confused by their education, often at boarding schools, which included the compulsory adoption of Christian names. The adults missed the freedom of their old life on the plains. They were left completely without hope.

# Helping you learn

## Progress questions

1. What is the meaning of these words:

(a) homesteader
(b) sod house
(c) chips
(d) dry farming
(e) reaper
(f) threshing machines
(g) wind pump

2. (a) What kinds of transport and communication were available before the railroad? See figure 7, page 97.
   (b) In what ways did the railroad transform life in the west?

3. Why did the great cattle drives come to an end?

4. What was agreed by:

   (a) The Fort Laramie Treaty, 1851
   (b) The Medicine Lodge Council, 1867
   (c) The Fort Laramie Treaty, 1868

5. What happened at:

   (a) The Battle of the Little Big Horn, 1867
   (b) The Battle of Wounded Knee, 1890

## Discussion points

1. How wild was the 'Wild West'?

2. What do you really think lay behind the conflict between the white Americans and the native Americans? *Study tip* – Think about a wide range of cultural differences including attitudes to the land.

## Practical assignments

1. Find out more about the colourful characters of the west on the internet. See the list of web sites at the end of this book.

2. Draw up a table to show ways and incidents by which (a) the white Americans provoked the native Americans, and (b) the native Americans provoked the settlers and the army. Decide, on balance, which side you feel was more to blame.

| Means of Transport/ Communication | Details |
| --- | --- |
| Stagecoach | A system of public transport by which people could travel by horsedrawn carriage. It made scheduled stops along the various routes. Journeys were slow and uncomfortable. The most famous company was **Wells Fargo**, which dominated the West. |
| The Pony Express | A relay of young horse riders, who carried messages on very thin paper from **St. Joseph, Missouri to Sacramento, California in ten days**. They changed specially chosen horses at the 157 relay stations along the 2,000 mile route. They averaged 75 miles per day. The service lasted just under 20 months, 1860-62. It was put out of business by the telegraph system. |
| The telegraph | A method of sending messages by electrical signals by wire. **Samuel Morse pioneered the first effective system in 1837**. In the early stages, it was only used over short distances but it gradually extended across the west. |
| The railroad | The greatest development in opening up the west. The most notable achievement was the first transcontinental railroad. The government provided generous grants of money and free land to the railroad companies. **The Central Pacific started eastward in Sacramento, California; the Union Pacific worked westward from Omaha, Nebraska. They met at Promontory, Utah, on 10 May 1869**. It was a stunning engineering achievement, which involved blasting tunnels through the Sierra Nevada Mountains and building a long series of bridges. It was built largely by Chinese labourers in the west and by Irishmen, Civil War veterans and ex-slaves in the east. There was a heavy loss of life. |

Figure 7. How improved communications opened up the West.

## 8

# Hitler's Rise to Power

*One-minute summary* – The Weimar Republic was set up after Germany's defeat in the First World War (1914-18). It died when Hitler became chancellor on 30 January 1933. Within 20 months he made himself dictator of a one party state. Hitler's rise to power is a complicated subject. It is important that you understand that there are two themes working side by side: the weaknesses and mistakes of the Weimar Republic, and Hitler's cleverness in exploiting these problems. It helps if you break the period 1919-34 into smaller units. As you study this chapter, make sure that you can explain:

► how the Weimar Republic was set up
► why the Treaty of Versailles was hated in Germany
► problems faced by the Weimar Republic
► the origins of National Socialism
► how Hitler appealed to different sections of society
► how Germany went from a Republic to a Nazi dictatorship

## How the Weimar Republic was set up

The German Federal Republic, 1919-33, is generally known as the 'Weimar Republic'. It is named after the town of Weimar where the first political assembly met. Berlin was threatened by revolution.

### Key dates
The key dates in the setting up of the Republic were:

9 November 1918    Kaiser William II abdicated.

11 November 1918    Germany signed the armistice with the allies. This ended the first world war which began in 1914

June 1919    The Treaty of Versailles was signed.

August 1919    The constitution of the Weimar Republic came into force.

There were two presidents of the Weimar Republic. Both died in office.

1919-25    Friedrich Ebert.
1925-34    Paul von Hindenburg – a First World War hero

The only democratic statesman of any real ability was Gustav Stresemann, chancellor (equivalent of our prime minister) in 1923, and foreign minister, 1923-29. His death in 1929 was a tragedy for the Republic.

# Problems faced by the Weimar Republic, 1919-23

The Weimar Republic was rocked by economic catastrophe and by a series of attempted revolutions. These nearly overwhelmed it in its first four years.

### Two built-in problems
It is important to remember that the Weimar Republic started with two very serious in-built problems:

1. It was unfairly blamed for signing the hated Treaty of Versailles, 1919. See figure 8, page 101.

2. The Weimar constitution 1919. This framework for government was very democratic in many ways. However, it contained two major flaws, which were to contribute to the downfall of the Weimar Republic.

    (a) The voting system, which was a form of proportional representation, led to a long series of unstable coalitions (government by two or more parties).

(b) Article 48 of the constitution allowed the president to rule by decree in an emergency. This gave the president the power to bypass the Reichstag (like our House of Commons). It was mis-used in the period, 1929-33.

▶ *Question* – Do you think that Germany had reason to be bitter about the Treaty of Versailles? See figure 8, page 101. Study tip: Answer the question in separate blocks. Some parts of the Treaty are more unfair than others. In terms of land, Germany was lucky not to be completely broken up, as the French had demanded.

## Threats from left and right

The Republic was threatened by revolution from the left and the right in this early period:

1. The Spartacists (the German Communist Party) tried to stage a revolution in January 1919. They were defeated by the Free Corps who murdered the Spartacists' leaders. Regional communist risings failed in 1920 and 1923.

2. Attempts to breakaway from the Republic to form independent states took place in several areas including Bavaria (1919) and the Rhineland (1923). These also failed.

These threats to the Republic were put down violently by the army supported by the Free Corps, which was disbanded in 1921.

(a) There was a series of political assassinations in this period. Murder victims included Matthias Erzberger, leader of the Centre Party, (1921) and Walter Rathenau, the Foreign Minister (1922).

(b) The Kapp Putsch, 1920. This was an attempted right wing state takeover led by Wolfgang Kapp, who wanted to overturn the Treaty of Versailles. The Putsch was put down by the workers who staged a general strike, which brought Berlin to a standstill. The army took no action.

▶ *Question* – What does the Kapp Putsch reveal about the loyalty of the army to the Weimar Republic?

| Germany's grievances | Details |
|---|---|
| 1. It was said to be a **dictated settlement** ('a Diktat' in German). | Germany was **not allowed to take part in the peace talks.** In effect, they were forced to sign the treaty. The only other option was to go back to war. |
| 2. **Germany lost** over 70,000 square kilometres of **land.** | In particular the Germans resented:<br>• the loss of the '**Polish Corridor**'. This strip of German territory was taken to give the newly created state of Poland access to the sea. This split East Prussia from the rest of Germany.<br>• The German port of **Danzig** became a free city administered by the League of Nations.<br>• Germany was stripped of **all her colonies.** They were redistributed between Britain and France as 'mandates'.<br><br>Germany also lost:<br>• **Alsace and Lorraine** to France. This was expected as Germany had taken these provinces from France in 1871.<br>• Small areas of land were also lost to Belgium, Czechoslovakia, Denmark and Lithuania.<br><br>On a temporary basis, Germany also lost:<br>• **The Saar coalfield**, was given to France for 15 years. This was to help compensate France for the grave damage that she sustained in the war. At the end of that time, the people of the area would vote on whether to return to Germany or to stay with France. |
| 3. **Germans felt humiliated** by the severe military restrictions imposed on them. | • **The army** was limited to 100,000 men. Conscription (compulsory enlistment) was forbidden. Tanks and poison gas were banned.<br>• **The navy** was limited to a total of 36 ships, this included a maximum of 6 battle ships. Submarines were forbidden.<br>• **The air force** was to be disbanded.<br><br>Germany was **forbidden to unite with Austria** (the 'Anschluss').<br>**The Rhineland** was to be a **demilitarised zone.** This meant that a strip of land 50 kilometres wide on the right bank of the River Rhine was to be completely free of military activity. Allied troops would occupy the area for 15 years. |
| 4. Germans were united in hatred of the '**War Guilt Clause**' (article 231 of the treaty). | **This clause said that Germany alone was responsible for the outbreak of the First World War.** This was felt to be totally unjust in Germany; other countries shared the responsibility. The clause was used to justify reparations. |
| 5. **The reparations (compensation) settlement** caused bitter resentment in Germany. It was the root cause of Germany's economic catastrophe in 1923. | • Germany said that she was forced to '**sign a blank cheque**'. This was because she had to agree to pay reparations in 1919 but the sum was not fixed until 1921.<br>• **The Reparations Commission fixed the sum at a massive £6,600 million.** Although this fell far short of the sum that the French wanted, Germany simply could not afford to pay the staged repayments. |

Figure 8. Why the Treaty of Versailles, 1919, was hated in Germany.

## What events led up to the crisis year of 1923?

1. Germany's reparations (compensation payments for the cost of the First World War) were fixed at £6,600 million in 1921.

2. In 1922, Germany paid the first instalment but announced that they could not afford to make any more repayments for three more years.

3. France and Belgium invaded the Ruhr in January 1923 to seize what they were owed from Germany's industrial heartland.

4. Germany responded by passive resistance. This meant refusing to co-operate with the invading forces in any non-violent way. As part of this policy, the Ruhr workers went on strike. They were paid by the German government.

5. The government soon ran out of money. It had been bankrupted by the war and was already crippled by the effects of the Treaty of Versailles. In desperation, it resorted to printing bank notes, which were useless because they were not backed by reserves of gold or other forms of security. This led to hyperinflation, when money completely lost its value. By October 1923, £1 was worth 10, 000 million marks. Money was literally not worth the paper it was printed on.

## What were the effects of hyperinflation?

1. Money became completely useless in Germany. Millions of marks were needed to buy basic commodities. However, the currency was so worthless, that people bartered for essential supplies such as food and fuel.

2. The middle class was hardest hit by hyperinflation. This was because they had salaries, which were paid monthly rather than weekly wages. Their savings and pensions soon became worthless. It was this class, which most lost faith in the Republic over this crisis. The rich were protected because they often owned land, which kept its value. The poor had no savings but they were hard hit by unemployment.

This crisis gave Hitler the perfect opportunity to stage his first attempt to seize power.

▶ *Question* – Why did Hitler hope that people might give up supporting the Weimar Republic and turn to him when he attempted revolution in 1923?

# What were the origins of National Socialism?

### Hitler's background

1. Hitler was born in 1889 at Braunau in Austria where his father was a customs official.

2. After an unhappy childhood, he went to Vienna hoping to be an artist. He failed in this ambition and lived in the city as a tramp from 1908 to 1913. This experience nurtured his anti-semitism (hatred of the Jews) as he blamed his failure on the Jews, many of whom had fled there from persecution in Russia.

3. Hitler volunteered to fight for the German army in the First World War (1914-18). He was awarded the Iron Cross (Germany's highest military honour) but was not promoted beyond the rank of lance-corporal.

4. In 1919, Hitler went to Munich where he joined a small political party called the German Worker's Party, which had been founded by Anton Drexler. Hitler soon took over the leadership and changed the party's name to the National Socialist German Worker's Party. It was popularly known as the Nazi Party.

### The original Nazi programme

The original 25 point party programme (1920) was designed to appeal to almost everyone in Germany. For example, the party called for:

1. the union of all Germans into a greater Germany
2. the abolition of the Treaty of Versailles
3. German citizenship to be limited to those of German blood – no Jew could be a German citizen
4. no more non-German immigration
5. nationalisation (state take over) of large industries
6. generous benefits for old age pensioners

▶ *Question* – Which of these points would have appealed to
(a) German nationalists, (b) the poor, and (c) all Germans?

▶ *Question* – When Hitler got into power, he dropped the socialist
parts of the programme because he wanted the backing of big
business. Which points would he have dropped?

## How Hitler appealed to different sections of society

### Hitler's ideas

The 25 Point Programme gives an insight into Hitler's thinking. Few
of his ideas were original but he repackaged them in a new way. He
believed that:

1.  Germany's defeat in 1918 was the fault of the 'November crim-
    inals', Jews and communists who had conspired with Germany's
    enemies to sign the armistice on 11 November. Germany could
    have won the war if she had not been 'stabbed in the back'.

2.  The Aryans (Germanic peoples) were the 'master race' because
    they had 'pure blood'. The Jews, the Slavs (east Europeans) and
    other people were said to be 'untermenschen' ('subhumans') who
    must no longer be allowed to 'contaminate' pure German blood.

3.  The master race was entitled to 'Lebensraum' ('living room') in
    which to settle their expanding population. They should expand
    at the expense of the 'Untermenschen'. Hitler was claiming the
    right to expand eastwards.

4.  German greatness should be restored. This involved the overturn-
    ing of the Treaty of Versailles and the union of all Germans in a
    Greater Germany.

▶ *Question* – Why do think that some of Hitler's ideas might have
seemed attractive to many Germans in 1920?

## The significance of the Munich Beer Hall Putsch

Hitler staged his first attempt to seize power in November 1923. He announced his plans to march on Berlin at a large beer hall in Munich on 8 November. He was supported by General von Ludendorff, who was a great hero of the First World War. The next day the two men and the SA (the Stormtroopers who were the paramilitary wing of the Nazi Party) marched through the centre of Munich. They were stopped by the police. Sixteen Nazis were shot.

*Hitler on trial*
Hitler and Ludendorff were tried for treason. Ludendorff was acquitted. Hitler used his trial to publicise his ideas. He was sentenced to five years in prison but served only nine months in the Landsberg prison, where he was treated very leniently. Hitler used the time to write a book, *Mein Kampf* (*My Struggle*), in which he explained his ideas on a wide range of subjects as well as telling his own life story.

▶ *Question* – Although the Munich Beer Hall Putsch was defeated, it was not a complete failure for Hitler. How do you explain this contradiction?

## Were the years 1924-29 a period of failure for the Nazi party?

The years 1924-29 were a period of stability for the Weimar Republic. The economy was settling down as a result of a new currency (the Rentenmark), loans from the USA and the Dawes Plan, 1924, which re-scheduled the reparations payments. These were further restructured by the Young Plan, 1929.

Thanks to Stresemann, Germany was being accepted once again by other countries. She signed the Locarno Treaty accepting her western frontier in 1925 and joined the League of Nations in 1926.

*Poor years for the Nazis*
On the surface, they were poor years for the Nazi party, which flourished in times of economic and social distress. Hitler used this lean

period to build up vital support in the police, army and big business and to consolidate party organisation. In particular he relied on:

▶ The SA (Sturmabteilung) also known as 'Brown Shirts'. They were thugs who broke up rival political meetings and were involved in street fighting. Ernst Röhm became their leader in 1930.

▶ The SS (Schutzstaffel) Hitler's elite bodyguard, who were also known as the 'Black Shirts'. They were physically and intellectually superior to the SA and were infinitely more dangerous. From 1929, they were led by Heinrich Himmler.

▶ *Question* – What does this planning show us about Hitler as a leader?

## How Germany went from a republic to a Nazi dictatorship

### From crash to depression

The situation changed completely in October 1929 with the Wall Street crash. The collapse of the US stock market triggered depression throughout the industrialised world.

In Germany, its effects were catastrophic. Germany was heavily reliant on US loans and on a small number of heavy industries, which were hardest hit by the depression. Unemployment in Germany soared from 1.3 million in September 1929 to over 6 million in 1932.

Hitler's promise of strong government and a revival of German national pride became increasingly attractive. This link between the economy and the support for the Nazis in the elections is clearly shown in the following chart.

| General election | Number of seats won by the Nazi party | Economic position |
|---|---|---|
| December 1924 | 14 | The economy had stabilised. The Dawes Plan rescheduled reparations payments. US loan of 800 million marks. |

.../cont.

| General election | Number of seats won by the Nazi party | Economic position |
|---|---|---|
| May 1928 | 12 | Economy still relatively stable. Unemployment: 1.3 million. |
| September 1930 | 107 | A year after the Wall Street crash. Unemployment: 3 million. |
| July 1932 | 230 | The depth of the depression. Unemployment: 6 million. |
| November 1932 | 196 | Unemployment began to fall. Unemployment: 5 million. |

▶ *Question* – When was Nazi support lowest? How do you explain this?

▶ *Question* – When was Nazi support highest? How do you explain this?

## Political events

1. Brüning of the Catholic Centre Party was chancellor, 1930-32. He pushed through pay cuts for government workers and increased taxes by using Article 48. Brüning called an election in September 1930. This allowed the Nazis to increase the their seats from 12 to 107. The moderate parties lost their seats as people turned to the extremists.

2. Brüning continued as chancellor with the backing of President von Hindenburg who used article 48 to issue emergency decrees. In the end, Hindenburg forced Brüning to resign in May 1932. The President had been influenced by General von Schleicher.

3. In April 1932, Hindenburg was re-elected with 19 million votes. Hitler stood against him and won 13 million votes. The communist candidate won only 3 million votes.

4. The new chancellor was Franz von Papen of the Centre party. He held another election in July 1932 hoping to increase his 68 seats. This gave Hitler the chance to become the largest single party in

the Reichstag with 230 seats. Hindenburg did not give in to Hitler's demands to be made chancellor. Another election in November 1932 further reduced Papen's support in the Reichstag, but so too did the Nazis'. This reflected a downturn in the unemployment.

5. Papen resigned and was replaced by General von Schleicher. He lasted only two months in office, and was the last chancellor of the Weimar Republic. He was brought down by a secret plot between Hitler and Papen: Hitler was to be chancellor; Papen was to be his vice chancellor. Papen believed that he would really be in control. Hindenburg agreed to this plan. Hitler became chancellor on 30 January 1933.

▶ *Question* – How important is Papen in explaining how Hitler came to power?

## Hitler's methods

1. He exploited the mistakes of the Weimar Republic.
2. He played on people's fears and prejudices.
3. He used brilliant propaganda orchestrated by Joseph Goebbels. This involved clever posters with clear messages, and huge rallies with the swastikas, marching music and stirring speeches.
4. He was a clever speaker, who used clear, simple messages, which were often repeated.
5. He used violence through the SA and SS.
6. He presented himself as Germany's 'last hope'.

▶ *Question* – Which of these methods do you believe are the most important in explaining Hitler's rise to power?

## How did Hitler move from chancellor to dictator, 1933-34?

When Hitler became chancellor he was in a politically weak position. There were only three Nazi ministers in the government and the party did not control the Reichstag. The president had the power to dismiss him and rule by decree. Hitler's first aim in government was to win total power. You need to know how Hitler managed to achieve this ambition by August 1934.

## The Reichstag Fire, 27 February 1933

This is a very important incident, which often appears on exam papers. The Reichstag building burned down a week before the election. Marinus van der Lubbe, a Dutch communist of very limited understanding, was found in the burning building. Historians argue about what really happened:

1. Was it really a Nazi plot masterminded by Goering and Goebbels to discredit the communists before the election?
2. Was it a communist plot?
3. Did van der Lubbe act alone as he claimed throughout his trial?

The evidence is not conclusive. There are many unanswered questions including: how did van der Lubbe get into the building? How did he get hold of the huge quantities of fire lighting materials involved? The importance of the fire is that it gave Hitler the excuse to:

(a) suspend basic civil liberties

(b) crush the Communist Party just before the election.

▶ *Question* – Which do you think is the most likely explanation for the Reichstag Fire?

> Study tip: Find answers to as many of the unanswered questions as you can.

## The election, 5 March 1933

The Nazis increased their seats from 196 to 288, but they still did not control the Reichstag. They achieved a majority by persuading the right wing Nationalist party to merge with them. That still left the Social Democrats, the Communist party and the Catholic Centre party, who continued to oppose him. Hitler disposed of this threat by passing the Enabling Law.

▶ *Question* – What do these election results suggest about the Nazis' support after just over two months in power?

## The Enabling Law, 23 March 1933

This act would effectively suspend the Reichstag for four years. The powers of the president and the elected assembly would pass to Hitler as chancellor.

Under the terms of the Weimar constitution, the act needed the support of two-thirds of the Reichstag because it involved a change in the way in which the country was governed. Hitler achieved this by intimidating use of the SA and the SS. Only 94 Social Democrats voted against it, so Hitler was able to do away with the Reichstag. He was now a dictator with no elected assembly to curb his powers.

Hitler wasted no time in eliminating all political opposition. On 14 July 1933 the Nazi party was declared to be the only legal party in Germany.

▶ *Question* – Why was the Enabling Act so important to Hitler's plans to take full control of Germany?

▶ *Question* – Why was the Enabling Act passed?

## How did Hitler achieve Gleichschaltung (co-ordination)?

The Nazis undertook a policy called 'Gleichschaltung' or 'co-ordination' to bring key elements in the state into line with their party between 1933-34. This involved:

1. the Länder (the 18 states of the federation) – Nazi governors were put in charge of each state

2. the civil service – all Jewish civil servants were sacked

3. the legal profession – all judges and lawyers had to be Aryan, Nazi supporters. People's courts were set up. They were really Nazi courts

4. the police were taken over by the SS. Himmler was in overall charge

5. the trade unions were replaced by the German Labour Front (the DAF). Strikes were banned.

## Why did Hitler stage 'the Night of the Long Knives', 30 June 1934?

Hitler still was not satisfied. He wanted to wipe out Röhm, the SA and other possible enemies in a surprise attack. He was prompted by:

1. Fear of Ernst Röhm, who wanted to merge the regular army (the Reichswehr) with his SA. Hitler and the generals feared the idea of a merger. Hitler did not want Röhm to become too powerful. The generals knew that the SA would swamp the regular army.

2. The knowledge that President Hindenburg would die very soon. Hitler wanted to make sure that his power base was completely secure before he made his final bid for total power.

On the night of 30 June 1934, Röhm was arrested and shot by the SS when he refused to kill himself. Many other SA leaders were also killed. In all at least 400 people were murdered by the SS including General von Schleicher. Hitler's gamble had paid off. He had eliminated Röhm, crushed the threat from the SA, and won the support of the generals at a crucial moment.

### The Führer

President Hindenburg died on 2 August 1934. Hitler immediately took over as head of state as well as head of government. He called himself the 'Führer' or 'Leader'. In fact, he was dictator of a one-party state.

# Helping you learn

### Progress questions

1. What two features of the Weimar constitution contributed to the downfall of the Republic?

2. What were Germany's main complaints about the Treaty of Versailles?

3. How were the following attempted revolutions put down:

   (a) the Spartacist rising, 1919
   (b) the Kapp Putsch, 1923
   (c) the Munich Beer Hall Putsch, 1923

4. Why was 1923 such a critical year for the Weimar Republic?

5. What were the key steps in

   (a) Hitler's rise to power, 1929-33
   (b) his consolidation of power, 1933-34

## Discussion points

1. Was the Weimar Republic doomed from the start?

2. Why did the republic survive in 1923 but fall in 1933?

## Practical assignments

1. Draw a timeline of events of the period, 1919-33 to show the key events in Hitler's rise to power.

2. Look up the events of 1929-33 on the internet. See the list of web sites at the end of this book.

# 9

# Life in Nazi Germany

*One-minute summary* – As soon as President von Hindenburg died on 2 August 1934, Hitler was dictator of a one party state, which he called the Third Reich or Empire. It was a 'totalitarian' regime. This meant that the government controlled every aspect of people's lives. In particular, you need to focus on:

▶ how the Nazis tried to indoctrinate young people

▶ how the Nazis tried to control the lives of women

▶ how the Nazis influenced culture

▶ Nazi policy towards religion

▶ the success or failure of Nazi economic policy

▶ the stages in the persecution of the Jews

▶ other minorities persecuted by the Nazis

▶ the impact of the Second World War on life in Germany

Once the Nazis were in power they were able to put their terrible racial and social policies into practice. You must understand how his staged persecution led to the Holocaust (the murder of 6 million Jews in Europe). Remember that gypsies and other minorities were victims of Nazi persecution, too.

It is also important to remember that not all Germans went along with the Nazis. There was a significant but fragmented opposition to the regime throughout its existence. You need to know who opposed Hitler and what became of them.

## How the Nazis tried to indoctrinate young people

The Nazis placed great importance on children and young people because they represented the future. They tried to indoctrinate (brainwash) them both in school and their leisure time.

### German schools

In school, children were subjected to non-stop indoctrination. Even the youngest children were taught to sing Hitler's praises. School timetables were re-drawn to reflect Nazi ideas. Religious Education disappeared. Children were taught the Nazi beliefs about race in a new subject called 'eugenics'.

All subjects were used as part of the indoctrination programme. Particular stress was placed on PE. This reflected the real purpose of education. Boys were destined for armed service for the Reich; girls were to be mothers.

▶ *Question* – How do you think that history, geography, and biology could be twisted to indoctrinate children in Nazi ideas?

▶ *Question* – Why do you think that Religious Education was dropped?

In order to carry out these policies the Nazis had to rely on the support of the teachers. Jewish teachers and those with left-wing views were quickly removed. Those who remained had to swear an oath of personal loyalty to Hitler. Teachers' unions were replaced by the National Socialist Teachers Alliance.

Special Nazi schools were provided for children who were identified as future leaders of the Reich.

### German universities

Nazi control of education extended to the universities. Jewish lecturers and those who would not co-operate were sacked. The Nazis did not encourage higher education and the number of higher education students fell under the Third Reich.

▶ *Question* – Why do you think that the Nazis did not encourage university education?

## Youth organisations

Out of school, the Nazis continued their indoctrination of children and young people through youth organisations. On the surface, they appeared to be harmless. They offered hiking, camping and outdoor activities of all kinds. Members wore uniforms and worked towards gaining awards in various skills. In reality, they were another method of brainwashing and preparation for adult life as planned by the regime. They were rigidly divided as follows:

| | |
|---|---|
| The Little Fellows | boys aged 6-10 |
| Young German Folk | boys aged 10-14 |
| Young Girls | girls aged 10-14 |
| Hitler Youth | boys aged 14 to 18 |
| League of German Girls | girls aged 14-18 |

These organisations were not entirely successful. Not all children joined, even after membership was made compulsory in 1939. A minority rebelled against the Nazi regime (see figure 9, page 124).

▶ *Question* – Why do you think that youth organisations might appeal to parents?

# How the Nazis tried to control the lives of women

The Nazi regime saw women's lives as limited to 'children, church and kitchen' (the so-called 'three Ks' from the initial letters in German).

### Motherhood

The principal role of a woman was said to be motherhood. Aryan women were encouraged to marry early, and to have as many children as possible by:

1. marriage loans which did not have to be repaid after the birth of the fourth child

2. generous child allowances

3. medals for mothers of large families

These policies failed to boost the birth rate as the Nazis had hoped.

### Women at home
Women were encouraged not to work. This helped to reduce unemployment. However, by 1938, there was a change in policy as the labour shortage was beginning to bite.

### Women's appearance
Women were discouraged from adopting up-to-date hair styles and fashions. These ideas were promoted by the Nazi Women's League. This organisation had only limited membership.

### Women and politics
It is important to note that women played no major role in the Nazi government.

▶ *Question* – How successful were the Nazis in controlling the lives of women?

## How the Nazis influenced culture

Culture was controlled by the Reich Chamber for Culture. Its head was Joseph Goebbels, who was Minister for Enlightenment and Propaganda. Under his direction, the arts were used to spread anti-semitism and to encourage conformity to what the Nazis considered to be social norms.

### Nazi cultural controls
1. Work of any kind by Jews or communists was banned.

2. Banned books were burnt in public by the SA.

3. Jazz and swing music was banned. There was a heavy stress on traditional German music by Aryan composers.

4. The press was tightly controlled and rigorously censored.

5. The radio was seen as a good means of propaganda.

6. Modern art was said to be 'decadent' and was banned. Artists

were encouraged to depict themes reflecting Nazi ideas of society and beauty.

7. The film industry was encouraged to spread propaganda messages.

8. Posters spread propaganda throughout Germany.

9. Many leading world class artists fled from Germany before Hitler came to power. As a result, artistic standards fell dramatically in Nazi Germany.

▶ *Question* – How successful do you think Goebbels was in controlling people's thoughts through his use of culture as a form of propaganda?

## Nazi policy towards religion

Nazism and Christianity are fundamentally opposed systems of beliefs. However, Germany was a strongly Christian country, and the Nazis tried to control rather than suppress Christianity.

### The Catholic church
Hitler made an agreement with the Pope in 1933. The Church agreed to keep out of politics in Germany in return for a promise of special protection for the position of the Catholic church in Germany. The Nazis soon broke this pact.

Pope Pius XI openly criticised the Nazi regime in an encyclical (letter) in 1937. Relations between the Catholic church and the Nazi regime deteriorated but the church was not systematically persecuted.

### The Protestant church
(a) The Protestant churches were easier to attack than the Catholic church, which was a world-wide organisation based in Rome. The Nazis tried to set up their own Protestant church. Ludwig Müller was its leader. He tried to square Nazi ideas with Christian teaching. Pastor Martin Niemöller led a breakaway church, which remained true to Lutheranism. The Lutheran

theologian Dietrich Bonhoeffer, was implicated in the July Plot, 1944 (see figure 9, page 124) and was executed just before the end of the war.

(b)  The Jehovah's Witnesses were victims of Nazi persecution.

(c)  The regime tried to start a pagan form of religion called the German Faith Movement. It had very little popular support.

▶  *Question* – How successful was the Nazis' attempt to control religion in the Third Reich?

## The success or failure of Nazi economic policy

### Economic aims
Hitler had two principal economic aims once he was in power:

1.  to reduce unemployment, which averaged 4.8 million in 1933

2.  to rearm Germany on a massive scale. This would allow German expansion, the achievement of a Greater Germany and 'Lebensraum'. Hitler was definitely thinking in terms of war after 1937, although he believed that the war would be a short one.

### Unemployment
The reduction in unemployment was achieved by a series of radical measures:

1.  Public work schemes provided mass employment on state funded schemes such as building schools, railways, bridges, houses and barracks. Most important of all was the building of 2000 miles of autobahnen (motorways) throughout the country.

2.  Young men and women aged 19-25 had to work for six months in labour camps, directed by the Reich's Labour Service (RAD). They were paid a pittance and were subject to military-style discipline.

3.  Conscription (compulsory enlistment in the armed services) was introduced for all young men in 1935.

4. After 1937, rearmament provided huge numbers of jobs directly in shipbuilding and armaments and indirectly in iron, steel and coal industries.

5. Women were encouraged to leave the workforce.

6. Jews and 'asocials' (see page 123) were forcibly removed from the work force.

▶ *Question* – Which two elements of this economic policy were illegal under the terms of the Treaty of Versailles?

These policies were successful. The unemployment figures fell dramatically:

1934   4 million<br>
1936   1 million

Before the outbreak of the war in 1939, Germany had a labour shortage of half a million workers.

**Four Year Plan**
The Four Year Plan was introduced in 1936 under the direction of Hermann Goering. Its aims were:

1. rearmament – the armed forces were to be ready for war by 1940.

2. autarky – economic self-sufficiency. Germany was to produce essential raw materials rather than continuing to rely on imports from abroad. This was a vital part of planning for war.

The plan had patchy success. Germany did produce her own synthetic oil and rubber under the plan but they were more expensive than foreign imports. The Hermann Goering Steel Works was built to produce steel from low grade iron ore, but it remained dependant on iron ore imported from Sweden. Heavy industry expanded under the plan. For example, between 1936 and 1938, steel production had increased by 3,000 tons.

**Food**

Goering also tried to make Germany completely self-sufficient in food. This even involved attempts to make artificial coffee. Home production of basic foodstuffs did increase but 17% of Germany's food was still imported in 1939.

## What was the impact of Nazi economic policy on the people?

*Industry*

The industrialists benefited most from these expansionist policies. They were awarded huge contracts for war-related work.

*The workers*

For the workers, the picture was more complicated. On the plus side:

(a)  Unemployment became a thing of the past.

(b)  Loyal Nazi workers were rewarded by subsidised holidays, even cruises, organised by the Strength Through Joy movement (the KDF).

On the negative side:

(c)  Pay levels were kept low and working hours increased.

(d)  There were no independent unions. They had been replaced by the German Workers Front (DAF), a Nazi organisation led by Dr Robert Ley.

(e)  Consumer goods were hard to obtain, as Goebbels believed in 'guns before butter'.

(f)  There was no freedom of movement for workers. They were not free to move jobs as they wished. Discipline was harsh.

▶ *Question* – In what ways did the Nazi economic policy (a) succeed, and (b) fail?

▶ *Question* – How do you think that the workers would have felt about these policies?

# The stages in the persecution of the Jews

The National Socialist Party had been violently anti-semitic from the very beginning. Nazi propaganda – masterminded by Joseph Goebbels – portrayed the Jews as rich, greedy, untrustworthy communists. The Nazis blamed the Jews for all Germany's problems, including defeat in the First World War. The Jews were a convenient scapegoat. In reality, there were only about 500,000 Jews living in Germany at the time of the Weimar republic. This was less than 1% of the total population of Germany.

### Early persecution

Once in power, the Nazis began a systematic persecution of the Jews, which culminated in the Holocaust, the mass murder of the Jews in Europe. However, it is important to note that the decision to carry out genocide (murder of a race) was not taken until January 1942. The main stages of persecution between 1933 and 1938 were as follows:

| Date | Act of persecution |
| --- | --- |
| 1933 | One-day official boycott of Jewish shops and businesses. Jewish civil servants were sacked. |
| 1934 | Jews were banned from the professions. |
| 1935 | The Nuremburg Race Laws: |

1. The Reich Citizenship Law stripped Jews and gypsies of their German Citizenship, which was limited to those of Aryan blood.

2. The Law for the Protection of German Blood and German Honour banned marriage or sexual relations outside marriage between German citizens and Jews.

▶ *Question* – What do you think was the real purpose of these laws?

.../cont

1938   1. 17,000 Polish Jews living in Germany were expelled from the country.

      2. Kristallnacht (the 'night of broken glass') 9/10 November. This was the real unleashing of organised violence against the Jews in Germany. It was revenge for the murder of an official in the German Embassy in Paris by a 17 year old Polish Jewish boy. All over Germany, Jewish businesses were looted and synagogues destroyed. About 100 Jews were murdered and 20,000 Jews were sent to concentration camps.

      3. Jews were banned from every kind of business. Jewish businesses were to be 'Aryanised' (taken over by Aryans).

      4. All Jewish children were expelled from school.

      5. Jews were banned from taking part in all forms of cultural and sporting activities.

---

1941 saw a turning point in the persecution of the Jews. In June of that year, the invasion of western Russia added more Jewish communities to those who had already fallen victim to Nazi Germany. The persecution of the Jews took a terrifying new turn:

1. All Jews over the age of six were ordered to wear the Star of David sewn onto their outer clothing.

   ▶ *Question* – What do you think was the purpose of this law?

2. At the Wansee Conference (January 1942) senior Nazis met to decide on the 'final solution'. This was the decision to kill every Jew in Europe. It led directly to the 'holocaust': the murder of 6 million Jews from Germany and occupied Europe. To carry out this horrifying act of genocide, special death camps were set up in remote places like Auschwitz in Poland. They had special gas chambers, which were designed to kill as many people as possible, as quickly as possible.

## Other minorities persecuted by the Nazis

Other minorities were persecuted because they failed to fit in with the Nazi blueprint for society. In particular:

1. *Gypsies* – were targeted because they were non-Aryans who were part of an international race, with its own language and customs. They lived a nomadic life and did not have permanent homes or jobs. Like the Jews, they were sent to death camps. About 11,000 were murdered at Auschwitz. Before the war, there were about 30,000 gypsies in Germany; only 5,000 survived the war.

2. *Physically and mentally handicapped people* – who could not make an active contribution to the state were subjected to euthanasia, so-called 'mercy killing'. The systematic murder programme started with babies and children. It was extended to adults in 1939.

3. *'Asocials'* – a diverse group who did not conform to Nazi ideas about how people should behave. They included tramps and the 'workshy', who were forced to participate in the government's employment schemes (see page 118). Alcoholics, prostitutes, homosexuals, criminals and juvenile delinquents were also classed as 'asocials'. They were sent to concentration camps, where many were forcibly sterilised.

▶ *Question* – Why were (a) the Jews, (b) the gypsies, (c) physically and mentally handicapped, and (d) the 'asocials' victims of Nazi persecution?

### The rise of Himmler's SS

In the early days the SA carried out much of the terror. After the 'Night of the Long Knives', 30 June 1934 (see page 111), the SA was eclipsed by the SS. Himmler built up a huge sinister empire, which included the:

1. SD – the party's police force, which was really an intelligence service
2. the regular police force
3. Gestapo – the secret state police, originally based in Prussia

| Opposition group | Details | Fate of the group |
|---|---|---|
| **Political opposition** | The Nazis smashed the communist and Social Democratic Parties, who offered the most resistance. All other parties were taken over by the Nazis, or agreed to disband, 1933-34. | Many leading members of opposition political parties were imprisoned. |
| **The Kreisau Circle** | A small group of officers and civilians who dreamed about rebuilding a Christian Germany after Hitler had been removed. They were thinkers rather than planners. | The Kreisau Circle was broken after the July Plot (see below). Many members of the group were executed. |
| **The Rote Kapelle** (the Red Orchestera) | A group of about 100 communist sympathisers, who operated a spy ring sending information to the Soviet Union. | The Nazis broke the network in 1942. Most of its leaders were executed. |
| **Religious opposition** | Martin Niemöller of the Confessional Church. Cardinal Galen spoke out against euthanasia. | Pastor Niemöller was imprisoned but survived, as did Cardinal Galen. |
| **Youth opposition** | The White Rose Group was a group of students based at the University of Munich. They circulated anti-Nazi leaflets. | Leaders Hans and Sophie Scholl (brother and sister) were executed. |
| | The Eidelweiss Pirates, a loose grouping of young rebels who fought the Hitler Youth and generally refused to co-operate. | Leaders were executed in 1944. |
| **Military opposition** (the July Plot, 1944) | The most serious threat to Hitler. Colonel Claus von Stauffenburg planted a bomb at Hitler's headquarters at Rastenburg on 20 July 1944. The bomb failed to kill Hitler. | Von Stauffenburg was executed as was anyone remotely linked to the plot. 180 to 200 people were put to death in revenge. |

Figure 9. Opponents of the Nazi regime in Germany.

4. Waffen SS – the fighting SS, which rivalled the army
5. Death's Head Units which ran the death camps.

A network of spies was set up all over the country to monitor everyone's movements. This network reached from Berlin to blocks of 30 to 40 houses.

### Opposition
Despite this high level of control, there was a significant but fragmented level of opposition to the Nazi regime.

▶ *Question* – Study Figure 9 on page 124. Why do you think that the Nazi regime was able to defeat opposition to its rule within Germany? *Study tip:* Think about (a) the network of control exercised by the SS, and (b) the fragmented nature of the opposition movement.

# The impact of the Second World War on life in Germany

In the early stages of the war (1939-45), German civilians were not hit too badly. This was because Germany's blitzkrieg ('lightning war') tactics led to a string of easy victories.

Hitler was anxious to make sure that disruption of civilian life was kept to a minimum, but this was not possible. There was:

1. increased taxation

2. rationing – which restricted civilians to a very limited diet, largely of rye bread and potatoes

3. women played an increasingly important role in war industries and in agriculture

By 1942, the tide had turned against Germany. The USA had joined the war and Germany was losing in North Africa and Russia. At home, Germany was subjected to increasingly heavy bombing.

### How was Germany affected by bombing?
The RAF (and the USAF after the entry of the United States into the war) bombed military installations, industrial centres and key cities.

The RAF bombed Berlin for the first time in August 1940, but the heavy bombing campaign did not start until 1942. Cologne, Hamburg, Berlin and Dresden were amongst major targets. About 130,000 people were killed.

### Germany's dead

When the war ended on 7 May 1945, Germany's war dead numbered 6.8 million. This included servicemen and civilians.

## Helping you learn

### Progress questions

1. Explain the Nazis policies towards: (a) young people (b) women

2. In what ways did Goebbels try to indoctrinate the mass of the people?

3. What were the main aims of Nazi economic policy? To what extent did the Nazis succeed in carrying them out?

4. Why and how did the Nazis persecute the Jews?

5. What other minority groups were persecuted? Why were they victims?

6. How did the Second World War affect civilian life in Germany?

### Discussion points

1. Did the Nazis succeed in gaining total control over every aspect of life in Germany? *Study tip:* consider the question of opposition.

2. Why did the Nazis succeed in carrying out the Holocaust?

### Practical assignments

1. Design a spider diagram to show the ways in which the Nazis influenced ordinary life in Germany. Make sure that you include: education and youth movements; womens' lives; work, leisure and religion.

2. Find out about those who opposed Hitler and his regime. For example: Dietrich Bonhoeffer, Pastor Niemöller, Oskar Schindler, and Colonel Claus von Stauffenburg.

This period of German history is the subject of innumerable films and books, both fiction and non-fiction. There are often documentary programmes about Nazi Germany on television, featuring original film footage of the period. You may find it helpful to use these resources to extend your knowledge and understanding of this subject. Books like Anne Frank's diary can heighten your awareness of the personal tragedies in the lives of individuals who suffered at the hands of the Nazi regime.

When reading or watching stories about life in Nazi Germany, always take care to distinguish between fact and fiction.

# Glossary

## Medicine Through Time

**anaesthetic** Drug which makes the patient unconscious.

**antiseptics** Substances which kill the bacteria responsible for infection of wounds.

**archaeology** The study of the past, involving searching or excavating for physical evidence.

**aseptic** Germ free. See also **antiseptics** and **sepsis**.

**bacteria** Germs.

**Black Death** The bubonic plague of 1347-50, a pandemic in which at least a quarter of the population of Europe died.

**bubonic** Relating to buboes or swellings.

**contagious** Catching, for example contagious diseases.

**crusade** A holy war.

**'dark ages'** A long period of decline in western Europe which followed the collapse of the Roman empire in the 4th century. The decline lasted until about 1000 AD.

**flagellation** A sign of penance in which people whipped themselves. This was to show God that people were sorry for their sins.

**gangrene** A deadly condition which causes tissue decay.

**humours** The ancient Greeks believed that people's physical wellbeing was governed by four humours (liquids): blood, phlegm, yellow bile and black bile. They believed that illness was a result of these humours being out of balance.

**inoculation** The practice of giving a person a mild dose of a disease.

**laissez-faire** A French phrase meaning 'leave things alone', often used when talking about social and economic policy.

**medieval** Of the Middle Ages period.

**miasma** A word used in Victorian times to mean 'foul air', thought to be the cause of diseases such as cholera.

**nationalised** Taken over by the state.

**pandemic** A mass epidemic, such as the Black Death.

**physician** A doctor.

**regressive** Backward, or backward-looking. The opposite of progressive.

**renaissance** A French word meaning rebirth. A great 'renaissance' affected all forms of European culture from about 1450.

**sepsis** Blood poisoning. See also **antiseptics**.

**sterile** (*medical*) Free of germs.

**surgeon** A doctor who carries out operations.

**trepanning**, or **trephining** Drilling holes in the skull. This ancient medical practice was probably connected with the idea of releasing evil spirits.

**utilitarian**. Someone in Victorian times who had a strong belief in efficiency and in the greatest happiness of the greatest number of people.

**vaccination** The practice of giving a person weak dose of germs to protect them from a particular disease.

**welfare state** A state which accepts substantial responsibility for the social care of individual citizens.

## The American West, 1840-1895

**cowboy** A cowhand or cattlehand.

**homesteaders** American farmers who benefited from the Homestead Act, 1862

**lynching** Hanging offenders without a trial.

**mandatory** Compulsory.

**massacre** A mass killing or mass slaughter.

**Mormons** Members of the Mormon religion, properly called the Church of Jesus Christ of the Latter Day Saints.

**nomadic** Leading a wandering life, with no fixed home.

**plains** Vast flat areas of land.

**polygamy** A marriage in which the husband has several wives at the same time. Polygamy was practised by the Mormons in America.

**ranching** The American word for raising livestock for market, such as cattle. A ranch was a large farm.

**rustling** The theft of livestock, especially cattle.

**shaman** A holy man who played an important role in native American communities.

**tipi** Tent covered by buffalo hide.

**trail** An unmade route across the countryside.

## Germany, 1919-1945

**Aryans** Germanic peoples.

**autarky** Economic self-sufficiency.

**boycott, to** To refuse to take part in something.

**coalition** A government made up of two or more parties.

**conscription** Compulsory enlistment in the armed services.

**genocide** The mass murder of a whole race of people.

**Holocaust** Mass destruction. The 'Jewish holocaust' refers to the Nazi's mass murder of millions of Jews in Europe.

**hyperinflation** An extreme form of inflation, when money completely loses all value.

**indoctrination** Brainwashing.

**Nazi** Short for 'National Socialist' in German.

**propaganda** Information which is designed or distorted to give a particular message.

**putsch** *(German)* An attempt to seize political power by force.

**republic** A state without a king or queen.

**scapegoat** A person blamed for someone else's problems.

**Spartacists** The German Communist Party after the First World War.

**totalitarian** A regime in which a government controls every aspect of people's lives.

# Web sites for GCSE History

The internet, or world wide web, is an amazingly useful resource, giving the student nearly free and almost immediate information on any topic. Ignore this vast and valuable store of materials at your peril!

The following list of web sites may be helpful for you. Please note that neither the author nor the publisher is responsible for content or opinions expressed on the sites listed, which are simply intended to offer starting points for students. Also, please remember that the internet is a fast-evolving environment, and links may come and go. You may find it helpful to use one of the search engines to locate these and other sites.

If you have some favourite sites you would like to see mentioned in future editions of this book, why not email the author, Mary Kinoulty, at the address shown below?

You will find a free selection of useful and readymade student links for history (and many other subjects) at the Studymates web site. Happy surfing!

Studymates web site:     http://www.studymates.co.uk
Mary Kinoulty email:     marykinoulty@studymates.co.uk

## Medicine

*The BBC*
http://www.bbc.co.uk/education/medicine/
The BBC has a tailormade interactive web site, specially for this GCSE course. Be sure to check it out.

*Spartacus Internet Encyclopedia*
http://www.spartacus.schoolnet.co.uk/
The Spartacus Internet Encyclopedia includes British history, 1750-1950. This provides a wealth of information. You will find sections

on poverty, health and housing (includes Edwin Chadwick); the emancipation of women (includes Elizabeth Garrett Anderson); and socialism and the labour movement (includes Charles Booth and Edwin Chadwick).

*The Black Death*
http://www.byu.edu/ipt/projects/middleages/LifeTimes/Plague.html
You can find out more about the Black Death by visiting this page.

*Edward Jenner and Vaccination*
http://www.sc.edu/library/spcoll/nathist/jenner.html
Information about Edward Jenner and the discovery of vaccination can be found here.

*The Florence Nightingale Museum*
http://www.florence-nightingale.co.uk/
Details about Florence Nightingale's life and work can be accessed here.

*St Thomas's Hospital and the Old Operating Theatre*
http://users.aol.com/museumweb/oothist.htm
Find out about St Thomas's Hospital and the Old Operating Theatre here. This site includes a virtual tour of the Old Operating Theatre.

*Louis Pasteur*
http://www.ambafrance.org/hyperlab/people/_pasteur.html
Some useful information on Pasteur is available here.

## The American West, 1840-1895

As you might expect, this unit is particularly well served by the internet, where there are so many American web sites. You can visit many exciting sites in America. This will give you an invaluable American perspective on American history.

*American History Sources for Students*
http://www.geocities.com/Athens/Academy/6617/west.html
You can find American history sources for students provided by

Global Access to Educational Sources at this Geocities page. This opens up many excellent links including:

*(a) The Westward Movement*

> Archiving the American West
> Early American Roads and Trails
> The Pony Express Home Station
> Wells Fargo
> The Oregon Trail (several sites)
> The Donner Party (several sites)
> The Interactive Santa Fe Trail
> The Mormon Trail
> Pioneer web sites (a great variety)
> Along the Chisholm Trail
> The Gold Rush (numerous sites)
> Links to the Mountain Men of the West
> The Museum of Westward Expansion
> The Wild West
> Women of the West Museum (a virtual museum)
> Terry's orders to Custer before the Battle of the Little Big Horn
>     Massacre at Wounded Knee, 1890
> The Native Americans

*(b) The Indigenous Peoples*

http://www.geocities.com/Athens/Academy/6617/indian.html
The same source on this native American page – has very extensive links on the Indigenous Peoples. These include:

> Native American Timelines (especially helpful on the Indian Wars)
> Native American Indian Resources
> The Native American Adventure
> National Museum of the American Indian
> Tribe Finder
> Native American Nations has information on individual nations
> Numerous sites provide general information native American
>     culture

*The Fort Laramie Treaty*
http://maple.lemoyne.edu/-bucko/1851_la.html
The terms of the Fort Laramie Treaty, 1851, may be found here. To view the later treaty, substitute the 1851 date in the web page address with 1868.

## Germany, 1919-45

*The BBC Modern World GCSE syllabus*
http://www.bbc.co.uk/education/modern/hitler/hitlehtm.htm
The BBC has a web site for the Modern World GCSE syllabus here. This includes detailed information on Weimar and Nazi Germany. This site has a link with the Anne Frank web site.

# Index

## Cultural Studies

A student's guide to culture, politics and society
Philip Bounds PhD

Most students of the Humanities/Social Sciences have the opportunity to take courses in Cultural Studies, either as an independent subject or as part of a syllabus in other areas such as Art History, Literary Studies and Sociology. This book meets the need for a concise introduction to Cultural Studies as it has taken shape in Britain. It is unique among introductory texts in combining themes, key writers and historical background to provide an excellent overview for students. Philip Bounds is a Lecturer in Cultural, Media and Film Studies.
*Studymates paperback 1 84025 125 5*


## The European Reformation

A student's guide to the key ideas and the events they shaped
Andrew Chibi PhD

Lecturers often lack the time to present this important subject as fully as students need. Students tend to be either blitzed with information unfamiliar to them, or presented with only the barest details, and expected to fill in the gaps themselves. Resource collections are limited and students often left out in the cold. Specially written by an experienced university history lecturer, this new **Studymate** presents the key facts of the European Reformation in a straightforward and student-friendly fashion to help the student understand very clearly the key reformers and their basic reforming principles. Complete with quick summaries and mini-tutorials, this book will meet the needs of lecturers and students alike.
*Studymates paperback 1 84025 130 1*


## GCSE English

The student-friendly way to winning higher grades in GCSE English
Michael Owen BA(Hons)

Universities and employers everywhere want applicants with good reading, writing, speaking and listening skills. That is why English is such an important GCSE to do well in. This Studymate starts with coursework and finishes with the exam; it gives lots of helpful tips and examples, showing how to improve your performance, gain better marks and achieve a higher grade. This book is specially for you if you are taking your GCSE in England, Wales or Northern Ireland; the syllabuses of all six examination boards are followed here. Michael Owen is an experienced teacher and GCSE English examiner. He is Head of English in a secondary school, and helps to train other English teachers. Most important, his methods really work. The number of his own students passing GCSE English with grades A* to C has almost doubled in recent years.
*Studymates paperback 1 84025 104 2*

## GCSE Sciences

Mastering the key topics in biology, chemistry and physics
John Guttridge BSc(Hons)

Many students struggle with science subjects at GCSE, finding many important topics hard to understand. The special appeal of this new book is to make these key topics crystal clear all so that even the most hesitant student will make progress. The easy language and learning level, illustrations, case studies and helpful exercises have all been carefully designed with the student's needs in mind. This new Studymate will be a real boon for thousands of candidates revising for the GCSE Sciences Double Award, GCSE Sciences Single Award, and the single GCSE subjects Biology, Chemistry and Physics.
*Studymates paperback 1 84025 119 0*

## Hitler & Nazi Germany

A concise study and revision guide for coursework and exams
Robert Johnson PhD, with a Foreword by Professor Jeremy Black

Are you studying twentieth century German history? Can you give a convincing account in discussion or essays of Hitler and Nazi Germany? How will you gather your evidence, and weigh the historical arguments? That's where this Studymate comes in. It will give you rapid access to the central themes, events and background, and to the key issues raised by this challenging episode of European history. You can use it as a study or revision guide, or as an effective starting point for your course. It is designed to help you build your skills as a history student, and improve your performance in essays, seminars, classes, and exams.
*Studymates paperback 1 84025 165 4*

## Practical Drama & Theatre Arts

A skills-based introduction for students, performers and technicians
David Chadderton

Concise, practical and readable, here is a really great introduction to the theory and practice of creating theatre. Written by an experienced teacher and practitioner, it is an ideal starting point for students, at school, college or in the wider community, wanting to gain the skills to succeed as performers, writers, directors, designers or technicians. Use this book to gain the ideas, experience and qualifications you need to succeed. David Chadderton BA(Hons) is based at the Mainstream Dance & Theatre Arts Centre in Manchester. He teaches open drama workshops and diploma classes, produces new courses, provides workshops, arranges liaison for schools, and is active on many drama and theatre projects. He also holds the City & Guilds Certificate in Further & Adult Education.
*Studymates paperback 1 84025 109 3*

## Speaking English
Handling everyday situations with confidence
Dorothy Massey BA(Eng) DipEd CertTESLA

Students living in Britain, or other English-speaking countries, need effective spoken English to enable them to handle everyday situations with confidence. This new handbook will provide students with all the vocabulary and grammar necessary to deal realistically and successfully with both formal and informal encounters, from giving personal and family information, to dealing with health matters, education, the workplace and other vital topics. This very practical book includes a glossary, useful addresses section, web sites for students of English, further reading section, and index. Above all this new Studymate reflects a diverse, changing and multicultural British society.
*Studymates paperback 1 84025 114 X*

## Studying Literature
A student's guide to reading and understanding literary works
Derek Soles PhD

A-level and first year university literature students will welcome this handy introduction to studying literature. Straightforward and very concise, it defines and describes the components of the major literary genres and of literary theory. It covers: the conventions of literary genres, sequencing of events, characters, the narrator, the setting, the message, metaphor, imagery and symbolism, the tone of writing, and the relevance of the author's life and reader's own perspective. It explains traditional analytic methods, and brings you right up to date with more theoretical approaches, too. Step-by-step it gives student-friendly explanations which will boost your performance in coursework and exams. Derek Soles BA(Hons) MA PhD teaches English literature at both undergraduate and postgraduate levels, and is author of *Lessons in Essay Writing* (Prentice Hall).
*Studymates paperback 1 84025 131 X*

## Studying Poetry
Key skills and concepts for literature students
Richard Cochrane BA(Hons) PhD

Do you need to write about poetry? Do you find it frustrating? Is it difficult to find much to say? In this book you will discover the key to understanding poetry, and the secrets which raise your grades in coursework and exams. This book shows you how poetry works and how to make sense of it. It's full of practical explanations of advanced ideas which will radically improve your performance as a student. It covers traditional analytic methods, and brings you right up to date with more theoretical approaches, too. The author takes you through all the main elements of poetry, fitting them into a step-by-step approach which you can use in any situation. Quickly accessible, packed with key examples, and written in a friendly down-to-earth style, this book will equip you with all the skills you need. Richard Cochrane gained a first class honours degree in English from Cardiff University, where he went on to gain his doctorate and become an Academic Tutor in English Literature and Philosophy.
*Studymates paperback 1 84025 146 8*

## Studying Chaucer
Approaching the Canterbury Tales
Gail Ashton PhD

This Studymate invites you to engage with Chaucer's major work, *The Canterbury Tales*. Whether you are new to Chaucer, or more expert, this book offers a practical and supportive framework of ideas upon which to base your own exploration. It discusses how the narrative structure is organised through individual narrators and the sorts of stories they relate, through several layers of narration, and through a chorus of voices that encourage intertextual and multiple readings. Then, through a detailed analysis of some of Chaucer's key themes, you are challenged to consider the nature of writing itself. Gail Ashton is a Teaching Fellow at the University of Birmingham School of English. She is the author of other works on Chaucer, and gained her doctorate in Medieval Literature.
*Studymates paperback 1 84025 166 2*

## Studying History
A practical guide to successful essay-writing, seminars, assignments and exams
Robert Johnson PhD

Are you taking a history course at college or university? Do you know what the examiners are really looking for today? Can you gather evidence effectively, weigh the historical arguments, and present a convincing case in person or on paper? That's where this Studymate comes in. It has been specially designed to help you build your critical and analytical skills as a history student. Follow the step-by-step advice in this practical guide, and discover how you can radically improve your performance in essays, seminars, projects, classes, and examinations. Robert Johnson is a graduate of Warwick and Exeter Universities. He is a successful history lecturer, tutor and course manager, and an active member of the Historical Association. He is also author of *Hitler & Nazi Germany* in the Studymates series.
*Studymates paperback 1 84025 171 9*

## Understanding Maths
A practical survival guide to basic maths for students in further and higher education
Graham Lawlor MA

Are you enrolled on an arts or social sciences course in further and higher education, or a training course for work? Do you find it hard to cope with fractions, percentages, averages, decimals, angles, area, volume, or other number and data-related work? Then this is definitely the book for you. Written by an experienced and sympathetic maths teacher, it will help you master all these important skills. Whether you are just starting at college or university, or a mature student, it explains in easy steps everything you need for successful number and data handling.
*Studymates paperback 1 84025 124 7*